Yoga

Fights Flab

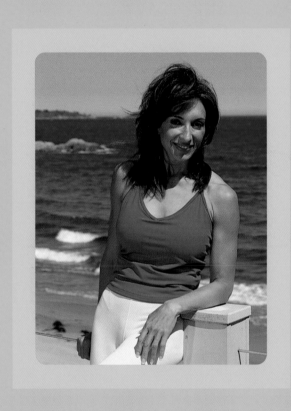

GLENDA TWINING

WITH ARNOLD WAYNE JONES

Yoga Fights Flab

A 30-DAY PROGRAM TO

TONE, TRIM, AND FLATTEN

YOUR TROUBLE SPOTS

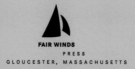

FAIR WINDS
PRESS
GLOUCESTER, MASSACHUSETTS

Text © 2004 by Glenda Twining

First published in the USA in 2004 by
Fair Winds Press
33 Commercial Street
Gloucester, MA 01930

08 07 06 05 04 1 2 3 4 5

ISBN 1-59233-058-4

Library of Congress Cataloguing-in-Publication Data available

Cover design by Mary Ann Smith
Book design by Yee Design

Printed in Singapore

The information in this book is for educational purposes only. It is not intended to replace the advice of a physician or medical practitioner. Please see your health care provider before beginning any new health program.

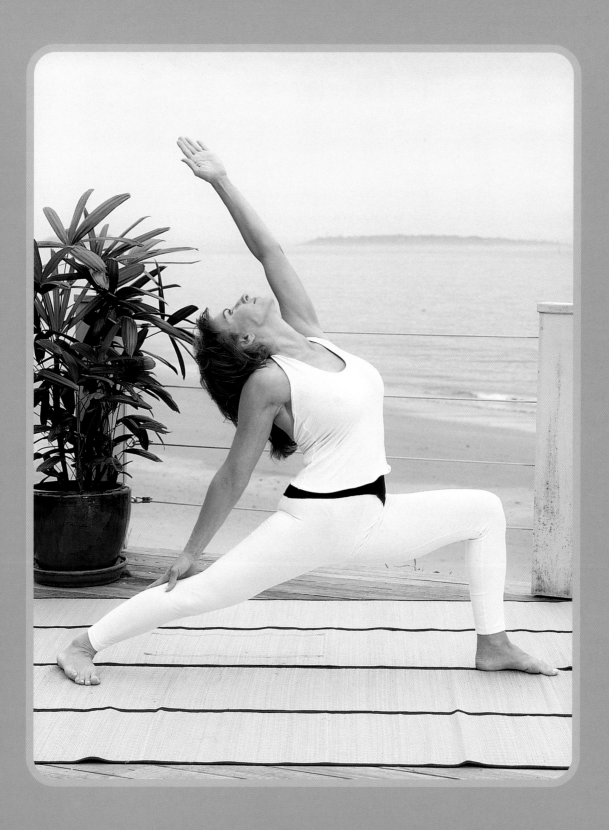

contents

A Flab-Free Reality

Consider this book your own personal invitation to a flab-free reality. Being overweight—flabby—is a concern and heartache for many people. We all want to be slimmer, to fit into a smaller clothing size, to look healthier, and to glow with an aura that comes only from mental and physical fitness. The issue is always how best to achieve this.

Of course, it is much easier to talk about losing weight than it is to do it. But with yoga, we don't have to just talk about getting into shape—we *can* do something about that!

I understand how difficult it can be to motivate yourself to take off those extra pounds, or even just to cut out that mouthwatering dessert. But the truth is, occasional exercise and fad diets will not have any lasting effect on your health. What you need is a *new* motivation altogether, something that does not take away from your life but adds to it.

So let's agree to take an entirely new approach to fitness and fighting flab—not thinking short term, but working on the positive elements of changing your life around. Let's do a 180-degree turnaround by approaching fitness as one of life's beautiful creations, based on compassion for the human spirit.

The secret, dear friends, is yoga.

THE FIVE YOGA ELEMENTS FOR HEALTH AND INNER PEACE

Yoga is a life of self-discipline that embraces simple living and high thinking. Ancient yogis regarded the body as a vehicle for the human soul. Just as a car needs gas, a good driver behind the wheel, oil for lubrication, a charged battery, et cetera, to function, so, too, the body has needs that must be met in order for it to function optimally.

The five elements to guide you in your quest for inner peace and achieving your goals are:

1. **PHYSICAL EXERCISE**. *One of the distinctive characteristics of yoga is that the physical exercises are not violent to the body, and provide gentle stretching to lubricate joints, muscles, ligaments, and tendons. These exercises, called asanas, will also provide toning and strengthening elements to keep the body in top physical condition. They are designed to do more than develop the physical body; they relax and strengthen the nervous system, facilitate circulation, and improve flexibility.*

2. **PROPER YOGA BREATHING**. *Deep breathing helps to clean and nourish the physical body. As you breathe in deeply, an abundance of oxygen is transported to every cell in the body. Deep exhaling expels waste products. Yoga breathing helps you relax in stressful situations, extends your physical endurance, energizes your body and mind when you are tired, and quiets your mind for peaceful rest.*

3. **POSITIVE THINKING, MEDITATION, AND VISUALIZATION**. *A balanced body and mind are essential for staying in control of your life. Regular meditation (or visualization) will help you achieve a clearer and more focused mind; positive thinking will result, which will purify the intellect. Positive thinking is the road that will take you to an experience of wisdom and inner peace.*

4. **EATING SENSIBLY**. *Everyone knows that various foods can have tremendous effects on the body, but they also affect the mind. Yoga, being so much about balancing body and mind, dictates that we have to be aware of what we consume. Simply put, eating wisely means staying away from junk food. This is not rocket science; it is common sense. You need to eat foods that are easily digested and promote good health—natural, wholesome foods—which will help you achieve a*

high standard of health, a keen intellect, and a serenity of mind. (This will be discussed in more detail in Chapter Three.)

5. PROPER RELAXATION. *When the body and mind are continually overworked and stressed, their natural efficiency is diminished. Studies have linked sleep deprivation or improper restfulness to everything from job-related accidents to decreases in reproductive fertility. Rest and relaxation are nature's way of giving the body a chance to recharge and increase its efficiency, including the burning of fat.*

My yoga program is probably unlike anything you've ever encountered. Too many exercise programs focus on negatives—a derivational approach to eating and fitness that works negatively. Yoga teaches us to focus on the positives: what foods you can eat to be healthier, what exercise routines will make you firmer, how to gain muscle and feel more alive in your body.

Yoga is not a cult or a religion; it is a lifestyle—one that comes with benefits greater than simply physical health. It aims for improving the total person. How many times have we heard of the "otherwise healthy" person dropping dead from heart disease, high blood pressure, et cetera, conditions that are too often exacerbated by stress? Being physically fit means very little if we don't approach living our lives as an affirmative experience in every particular. There are many factors that are encompassed in a decision to reshape one's life for the better. All of the chapters in this book are intended to guide you, step-by-step, in the quest to achieve the dream of a strong, fit, flab-free body.

☞ Join me as we increase your activity level and boost your energy … sculpt your muscles by strength training … work out even when you think you have no time … exercise mindfully and with purpose … become more flexible by stretching … achieve a healthy weight for you … and become body confident. And together we will learn how to keep the stay-motivated sizzle.

☞ Join me in becoming more positive and optimistic by soothing stress and developing healthy habits … developing a healthy mind … learning how to take time to nurture yourself and do more than survive. We can learn to tune in to our bodies and our hearts and nourish them in ways that are good for us. True fitness requires a holistic approach for optimum health and well-being, no matter what size or shape we are in.

☞ Join me as we approach sensible eating as the key to becoming leaner and healthier.

Ready, set, go! My amazing Total 30-Day Flab-Burning Program will guide you through a month of solid fat-burning training, including practical flab-fighting tips you can use on a daily basis. Best of all, you will learn how to maintain your new figure. With determination you can make it … and you won't believe it when you see the results!

HOW TO USE THIS BOOK

The chapters in this book are divided in such a way as to make your yoga experience an enjoyable one, and to make finding answers to specific questions easy.

Chapter One takes a look at body fat and what we can do to control it. Chapter Two discusses the body's metabolism in losing body fat. It is important to understand how we get flabby in order to fight it. This chapter includes secrets on how to keep fit. Chapter Three is about eating sensibly. This is not a diet book, but an understanding of how to use nutrition as part of your yoga regimen is essential. Chapter Four is about how emotions can affect us adversely, and what we can do to reverse those negative thoughts and increase overall health. Remember, practicing yoga is as much about spiritual and mental health as it is about physical health.

Chapter Five contains my Total 30-Day Flab-Burning Program. This is where you will find all the photos, instructions, and poses you need to know in order to fight flab. Follow this program, and you are on your way! Chapter Six features testimonials as well as some words and thoughts to help encourage and inspire you.

CHAPTER 1

Why You Need to Get Fit

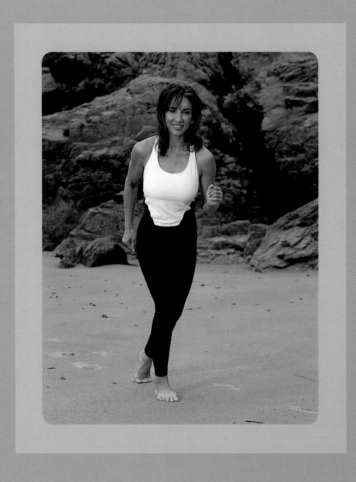

The human body is a remarkable machine. Its natural state is one of harmonious interaction between the physical, mental, and spiritual. Our bodies know a lot more about themselves than we often give them credit for. They are also far more versatile than modern living usually lets them be.

Take fat. Everyone needs fat on his or her body and in his or her diet. It serves as a barrier against the cold and stores up reserves of fuel in emergency situations. Each person's individual metabolism requires a different amount of fat, and every body stores fat in a different way. Some of us carry fat on our hips, and some of us carry it on our bellies. And some of us have it evenly distributed all around us!

The body does not, however, need *flab*. Flab is not fat; it is *excess* fat. And excesses of any kind can be dangerous.

HEALTH RISKS ASSOCIATED WITH BEING OVERWEIGHT

Data from the National Health and Nutrition Examination Survey indicate that nearly 65 percent of Americans were overweight and more than 30 percent were classified as obese in 2000; in 1980, only 46 percent were overweight and 14 percent obese. And the trend is toward even greater weight problems every single year. Children are increasingly obese; the costs to society in terms of lost work and health-related problems reach into the billions of dollars. Flabbiness has become nearly epidemic, and it is exacting a high cost in every aspect of our lives.

FLAB FACTS

The reason people become flabby is very simple: Food is taken in at a greater rate than it is burned off. When we eat excess food, we need to expend more energy to maintain the same weight.

When we don't burn off the excess calories we eat, those calories get stored in fat cells in the adipose tissue, just beneath the skin. When our used energy is too little and we take in more food than our bodies can handle, the fat cells get full and the cells divide to form new cells to get ready to be filled.

In the meantime, as we age, our muscles become less lean—and we become less active—which means we burn fewer calories over the course of a day and our nice tight muscles become loose and hold our figures differently. At the same time, few of us stop eating as much as we used to, which means we're adding more fat onto our bodies just as we need fewer calories to survive.

So, basically, we eat too much, we move too little, and our bodies change as we get older: That's how we get flabby.

Clearly, putting on flab pounds is a vicious cycle that feeds, so to speak, our body's dependence on fat. Eating less isn't the only answer. The body also needs to burn off the fat that is already stored.

Besides cutting calories by eating less and differently, the best way to lose flab is to create muscle. Muscle helps you burn fat, because the muscles are live tissue and need fuel to grow. They receive a portion of their fuel from the fat stored in your body. As you continue to exercise aerobically and do resistance training, your muscles grow, and they'll need more fuel, and they'll get that fuel from the fat cells. And that's how you lose weight.

Muscle also takes up less space than fat. Now, we're not talking about men who train to get bigger. That's one type of muscle. Women and men who do yoga will find that their bodies, as they lose fat, will take up less space and have a more lifted, leaner look because muscle is denser than fat tissue. A pound of muscle takes up less space than a pound of fat.

In fact, you can be flabby and not really fat. The amount of body fat you carry is much more important than your weight. Have your fat percent checked with a trainer or your doctor. For women, normal body fat is 20–25 percent of your body weight. For men, normal body fat is 13–18 percent. Anything over these percentages of body fat would be a fairly good indicator of the added risks of carrying too much flab.

THE SPECIAL PROBLEM OF CELLULITE

We know how many people—mostly women, but men as well—struggle with the unsightly and annoying fat known as cellulite, the lumpy fat sometimes found around the hips, buttocks, and thighs. Many of my students ask me for my help in getting rid of cellulite. It is a big deal for some women, who have tried everything from potions and creams to body wraps with negative results.

Some areas of our bodies have more fat cells than other parts. For example, on your forearm there will be relatively fewer fat cells than, say, in your hips; this is due to the larger capacity of fat storage in this area.

WHAT IS IT?

There is no special tissue that is called cellulite—it is only the name given to a soft, unattractively textured skin surface. It is the result of two factors: too little muscle and too much fat. The underlying muscle layer becomes too thin and the overlying fat layer becomes too thick. Without a firm foundation for the skin, it takes on the lumpy look of the formless fat layer beneath it. You do not even have to be overweight to have cellulite—just have more fat than muscle in a given area.

HOW DO WE GET IT?

Leading a sedentary lifestyle is a chief cause of cellulite. When we sit a lot, the hip and thigh muscles are the first to atrophy. Since most women carry their fat storage below the waist, with little muscle to support it, the skin's underlying foundation loses its firmness and the skin assumes the loose and lumpy foundation of the fat layer beneath it.

HOW DO WE GET RID OF IT?

The best way to fix cellulite is to strengthen and tone the muscles underneath the fat, according to a variety of studies. Once the muscle is strong and lean, the skin and the fat tissues near it will smooth out and the look of the cellulite will be changed. It may not go away forever or completely, but it will be much improved. The lack of strong muscle is the reason even thin women can have cellulite: it's because they don't have the proper muscle tone to hold on to their skin and fat.

For years I have sympathized with people, especially women, who battle cellulite, and after many years of teaching and studying, I have realized that it isn't pure luck that I do not have cellulite or show any sign of it, but it is directly related to the muscle tone I have maintained through the years, day in and day out, and also a result of the pure and healthy diet I have enjoyed for many years. Rebuilding muscle tissue makes you look better, feel better, and function better.

Research has indicated that a program of strength and endurance exercise combined with sensible eating can add about two to three pounds of muscle to your body and eliminate seven or eight pounds of fat after just about eight weeks. Because this program is intense strength training, it helps keep cellulite from becoming a problem. I am happy to say I have documented many of my students' results, and after a short eight weeks—or longer, depending on the time they allocate to their workout—the results were incredibly positive. Yoga offers particularly good resistance training in a low-impact format. While you might not be able to rid yourself completely of cellulite, you can make far more progress than if you just do nothing!

Hopefully this will help you understand the fundamental concepts of cellulite reduction and prevention—the sooner you start, the better!

THE SIMPLE TRUTH

Despite all the media attention lavished on diet pills, creams, different and expensive equipment, and "the magic diet," there are really only two ways to change your body shape. Any health professional will tell you exactly this. Simply:

EAT LESS AND EXERCISE MORE

Eating less does not mean you have to starve yourself—regular meals with nutritious food choices are outlined in Chapter 3, "Eating Sensibly."

If you regularly use up lots of calories through exercise, especially the balanced program outlined in the Total 30-Day Flab-Burning Program, where cardio and strength training are combined with stretching for more strength gains and maximum calorie burning, you will find your body becomes leaner, with fewer calories being stored as fat. You will boost your metabolism by increasing the rate at which calories are burned, and the result will be a fitter, stronger, and shapelier body.

IF YOU STILL DON'T BELIEVE YOGA CAN FIGHT FLAB…

Maybe you still have some doubts that yoga can fight flab the way I say it does. After all, how can a low-impact, solitary activity without any free weights or equipment other than a mat and towel take off the pounds?

You don't have to believe me, but you should believe Dr. Conrad Earnest of the Cooper Institute Exercise Physiology Lab at the nationally famous Cooper Aerobics Center in Dallas, Texas. I commissioned a special independent study of my yoga program to evaluate the activity levels of one of my yoga classes to prove that yoga fights flab.

Dr. Earnest took three test subjects—one of low physical fitness, one of moderate fitness, and one of high fitness (myself). He tested three major indices of exercise effectiveness: heart rate response, oxygen consumption, and caloric consumption.

A typical resting heart rate is 60–90 beats per minute; the average rate for those in the study was 145–150 beats per minutes, with some higher spikes twenty-five minutes into the class. So even though you stay in a small area for most of the program, you really get that heart pumping!

Dr. Earnest calculated oxygen consumption in several ways, noting that the most relevant was by determining the Metabolic Equivalent Units (METS), which allows comparison of one activity to another. The average METS for the test subjects was 4.7, with the highest being 5.5. "Moderate" activity occurs anywhere from 3.0–5.0 METS, and "hard" activity 5.1 and above. But the report went on to say that "the accurate measurement of more difficult tasks involving muscle strength … is not possible to do," so METS consumption was "likely underestimated by 12–15 percent. Therefore, even though your program is reported as Moderate Activity … it probably more accurately falls into Hard Activity." That means that practicing this yoga program is the equivalent of hard activity—a fact that is probably surprising to most who have not practiced yoga in the past, but not to those of us who are deeply involved in it.

The caloric consumption was equally telling. Dr. Earnest reported that the average total of calories burned was 5.4 per minute, or 324 calories per hour. For a 150-pound-person, that means my program burns more fat than an hour of calisthenics, or cycling at more than five miles per hour, or walking at more than three miles per hour, or swimming at a rate of twenty-five yards per minute. (One of the participants in the study burned calories at a rate of 381 per hour—that's almost as many as are burned in an hour's worth of tennis!)

Now do you believe yoga can make you slimmer and really trim that flab?

CHAPTER 2

Your Ideal Workout

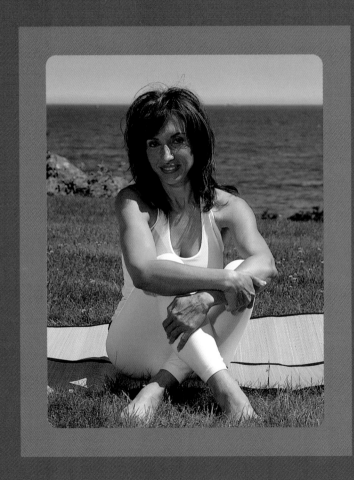

As important as it is to be flab-free and have a tight body, it is far more important to obtain a good fitness level. The term "fit" implies exercise and health, but also feeling comfortable in our bodies and having an abundance of energy.

This workout will physically and mentally prepare you to better deal with anything in your life. It will build your confidence and strength—when you are done, you will find that you are in the best shape not only for your body, but for your spirit as well. With determination you can make it—just wait until you see the results.

It's only too late if you don't start!

THE FIVE PHASES OF FITNESS

The body is designed as a phenomenal, useful machine to carry us through our lives of seventy, eighty, or more years. The skin and hair protect us and keep us warm, the skeleton and muscles protect our organs, and the brain gives us the intellect and intuition to avoid certain dangers.

But sometimes we make choices with our brain that are not good for our body, that do not aid in protecting us and keeping us healthy. Modern living has also infringed on the body's good sense with far more processed food and a much more sedentary lifestyle than nature intended.

But we cannot think of ourselves as victims of our environment or happenstance. Although heredity gives each of us different raw materials to work with, almost anyone can become fit with the right attitude and discipline.

Psychologists will tell you that as human beings, we go through stages as we come to certain understandings. You have no doubt heard of the five stages of grief: denial, anger, bargaining, depression, and acceptance. Well, in much the same way, we have to prepare ourselves psychologically to be fit. Here, then, are the Five Phases of Fitness, the steps we must go through in order to commit to being healthier and happier.

1. **MAKE A DECISION TO GET HEALTHY.** As a matter of fact, it takes only three or four seconds for you to decide you want to be fit, but, really, making a decision is more complicated than that—you need to make being healthy a habit. It takes three to four weeks for something to become a habit. My

program is designed with that fact in mind—it is a thirty-day schedule that, if you stick with it, will not only yield physical results within a month, but will create a new attitude inside you. Staying healthy will become your new habit. If you want to become fit, lean, and healthy, you will find every possible way to fit exercise into your schedule. Always remember: *Anything is better than nothing!*

2. **DON'T DOUBT YOURSELF.** It is absolutely natural to have doubts about any new undertaking, especially something that may seem foreign to you, like yoga. Although many of the practices in this book have been around for thousands of years, Western cultures really began to embrace them only in the last century, so they are not as ingrained in our psyches as traditional sit-ups or the 100-yard dash are. Add to that how exercise can lead to some initial disappointments if you don't see immediate results, and the potential for disappointment may be great. What you need to realize is that self-doubt is a natural part of the process of becoming fit. Face it— and move on! Even athletes doubt themselves, but those who conquer doubt are the success stories. *Make a decision to be one of the success stories.*

3. **CONQUER ANY DOUBT.** I make conquering doubt a separate step from the cognitive knowledge that you should not doubt yourself. That's because almost anything can be conquered if you truly set your mind to it. A central lesson of yoga is that once you make the decision to do something, you must do it physically, and doing that thing physically, increases your mental resolve! The human will can be a very powerful force; this is where the body and the mind connect. Exercising your body gives you the stamina and endurance to exercise your mind, spirit, and relationships with others around you. *Once you have made the decision, resolve to see it through.*

4. **TAKE YOUR HEALTH AND FITNESS SERIOUSLY.** Once you become fit, you will feel comfortable in all sorts of settings with all sorts of people. Your self-confidence will increase and open doors for you that you never imagined. Eating healthy will become a habit for you—fast food doesn't make you feel good, it just tastes good. *Know the difference.*

5. **SET AND ACHIEVE GOALS FOR YOURSELF.** Setting and achieving a goal provides tremendous satisfaction. When you complete this program after one full month, followed by maintenance three to four times a week, you will undergo a complete transformation. You will know you are fit, and you'll feel great! This program will definitely get you into top physical condition, but more importantly, the unbelievable amount of confidence you will gain in your abilities will change your life. The program is progressive, going step-by-step. It will help you realize things you may have thought impossible. You will feel energetic, alive, and confident. (There's a reason we talk about "building" confidence—it does not appear full-blown one day, but must be constructed like a fortress wall. Each brick may seem insignificant on its own, but together the individual bricks form a mighty structure. Build your confidence brick by brick, and you, too, will have the strength to do anything.) This workout program won't automatically give you confidence, but it will help you find the confidence within yourself, the same way it helps you build your strength and stamina through the fat-burning exercises. *Build your confidence.*

BUILD MUSCLE TO BURN FAT

In order to build muscle, you have to work the muscle through resistance training or weight-bearing exercise as we do in every upper- and lower-body yoga posture outlined in the program.

Some people don't see how yoga builds big muscles or reduces fat because they have been influenced by standard ideas of fitness—weight lifting makes your muscles grow, jogging gives you cardio strength to burn fat, et cetera.

What people fail to realize is that yoga does include weight lifting, only we are not lifting free weights but our own body mass. We get cardio activity through the breathing exercises and nonstop movement. Our muscles provide their own resistance, and when we work them, they siphon off energy from every cell in the body. Fat is replaced by muscle—simple as that.

THE VALUE OF A HEALTHY METABOLISM

Everyone has a different metabolism—the rate at which our bodies work through their internal mechanisms. Some people seem to eat and eat, never exercise, and stay thin as a rail; some can eat a scoop of ice cream one day and see it on their thighs the next morning. People's bodies differ, and we all have to accept that our body will behave differently from others'.

Even if you have a slow metabolism now, you can increase it by performing this thirty-day program. A *naturally* slow metabolism is no more a lost cause than a naturally slow runner is—with work, speed will improve.

The level of exercise produced by this program, when followed on a daily basis initially and then on a maintenance schedule of three to four times a week thereafter, *will* result in burning fat, with amazing results. Not only will you increase your metabolism while you are awake, but the efficiency of your systems will carry on even when you are asleep.

One of the key ways to increase your metabolism is to increase your muscle mass at any age—reduced activity will mean reduced muscle mass, which results in reduced metabolic rate. Build muscle to increase your metabolism to burn the fat!

THE SUPER-EFFICIENT WORKOUT TO BURN FLAB

My program is based on a very simple system made up of three exercise components:

Walk

Run

Yoga

Most athletes and fitness professionals will tell you that you need to walk before you work out, to prepare the body. Adding running and walking at the beginning of your yoga routine for the day is a matter of choice, but it is one I thoroughly recommend.

Although walking briskly is an equally demanding workout, you want to warm up the body completely and get your metabolism primed to burn fat.

Whether you choose to walk or walk and run is really a matter of personal choice. Both help in burning calories and getting you into the mood, and they both build up your aerobic activity before you start your yoga routine. The goal is increased fat burning from strength training and stretching for an overall body workout.

SCULPTING YOUR MUSCLES THROUGH YOGA

In almost every yoga posture, you are actually lifting weight—the weight of your own body. You lift, pull and push, and balance your body's weight, and as a result, you incorporate anaerobic exercise into your power yoga workout. Anaerobic exercises are muscle-strengthening, toning, and sculpting powerhouses, and combining this element with stretching or flexibility training will give you some of the most intense fitness and fat-burning benefits to be found in any exercise program.

The yoga poses outlined in this program are strong anaerobic exercises that strengthen, tone, and sculpt all specific muscles: Upper body, lower body, abs, and back.

Diligent stretching is as important as strength training and cardiovascular workouts in terms of achieving fitness and strength. The stretching, coupled with the yoga postures outlined in this program, will increase flexibility in your joints, muscles, and connective tissues. The stretching and counterstretching movements of these yoga routines will help you maintain balanced progress for increased strength and flexibility, working major joints and muscle groups.

SEVEN SECRETS TO KEEP FITNESS FROM FIZZLING

The greatest hurdle in achieving a flab-free body is losing enthusiasm for the workout. It's hard! I know. If it weren't, everyone would be thin and well muscled. But as John F. Kennedy so memorably stated in another context, we do not take on a challenge because it is easy; we take it on because it is hard.

1. **BE CLEAR ABOUT YOUR GOALS.** Know what your goals are *before* you begin your program. Write them down. Keep them handy. As you practice each pose, keep telling yourself that you can get into shape and get rid of the flab, that you can accomplish this, and how this will improve your life— you will be less tempted to skip a workout.

2. **PLAN.** The easiest way to lose the real benefits of this program is to make an excuse for why you need to cut a day here or a week there. The temptation will be great, but trust me on this—if you don't make excuses and you follow through, you will achieve more than you probably even imagined. The secret is to make a plan and stick with it. With your calendar in hand, find a place on every day for the next month on your schedule when you *know* you will have the little amount of time needed to sculpt your body. If you cannot do it at the same time every day, then alternate times—early in the morning before the kids are up, right before bed while your spouse is occupying the bathroom, during your lunch hour, instead of watching that rerun on TV. You do have the time, but you need to make practice a priority. Schedule your yoga workout sessions every day for the first month and four times a week thereafter—these sessions are just as important as appointments that cannot be missed.

3. **HAVE PATIENCE.** Don't expect to accomplish everything the first day or week—if you stay true to the program, your body will respond and you will see results quickly. Practice with patience and you will succeed.

4. **BELIEVE THAT CHANGE IS POSSIBLE.** Success derives from believing that you have control and that you can make something happen. Belief is more than just having a positive attitude. You *will* lose weight if you commit yourself to this program, and that knowledge makes the process exciting and possible.

5. **PRACTICE YOUR YOGA SESSIONS WITH LOVE AND COMPASSION.** We all like to reward ourselves—by sleeping late on weekends, by indulging in a pint of Haagen-Dazs, by curling up with a good book when the family is out of the house. Well, if you practice it correctly, yoga can be a reward as well.

Your sessions can be something very special, something you look forward to, something you love doing for yourself. Yoga can become your passion, your way of nurturing yourself.

6. **HAVE FUN.** Exploring and trying new things fuels the human spirit. Look on this undertaking as an adventure. There are many different routines in the program—enjoy them and have fun. Believe me, I don't like to get bored any more than anyone else does, so I have put together this program specifically to add vibrancy and diversity to each day's workout. There is enough variety to prevent boredom, which is usually the ultimate motivation killer.

7. **VISUALIZE YOUR SUCCESS.** As you will learn in Chapter 4, important components of yoga are meditation and visualization. If you think positive thoughts and visualize yourself accomplishing and succeeding even before you actually do it, you really are well on your way. Positive visualization is a tool used by many great athletes, and is crucial in making your program a success.

CHAPTER 3

Eating Sensibly

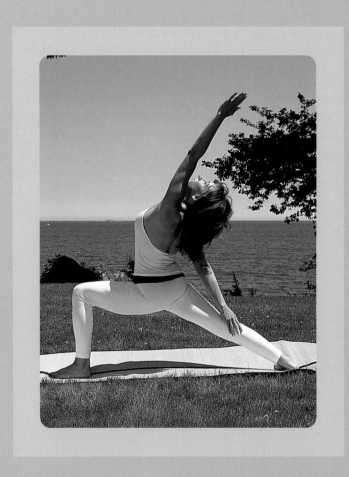

For most practitioners, yoga is not just exercise but a lifestyle. That means there is more to experiencing yoga at its fullest than simply working out for half an hour a day. You must approach your commitment to fitness as a complete way of living your life as a healthy person.

As part of this commitment, many yogis are vegetarians. I myself have been a vegetarian for thirty-five years and a vegan for twenty years. This is my choice; that does not mean it has to be yours. In fact, some of my best friends are meat eaters! I am not critical of them for their decision to be omnivores. I may have never considered, years ago while growing up in South Africa, that I would one day be living with my cattle-ranching husband in Texas, but that's where I find myself, and I love it.

If you are a vegetarian, or choose to become one, good for you. But if you are not, that's great, too. The only kind of eater you need to be is a smart eater.

"Eating sensibly" are better key words for losing weight than is the word "diet," which sets us up for failure. "Diet" automatically means deprivation and sets us up for a yo-yo effect of too much and/or too little. It is far better to create a lifestyle eating plan based on nutritious and delicious foods, as outlined below, featuring what to eat more of or less of to become leaner and healthier.

THE KEYS TO HEALTHY EATING

Any yoga program will naturally stress sensible eating as part of the philosophy of staying fit. Mine is no exception. The fact is, proper nutrition and diet will undeniably aid you in your goal to lose the flab. I do not propose a particular diet, but here are some pieces of good advice for fighting fat the yoga way.

EAT LESS AND MORE OFTEN

As I have frequently said, the body needs fuel in everything it does, whether running a marathon or stitching a hem on a skirt. Your body burns what is available, and because fat is stored in reserves, the longer you go without eating, the more your body feels deprived of energy. Worse yet, if you are engaging in any strenuous activity, your body may burn off muscle in order to power itself.

Shorter periods between eating, and consuming only what you need, keep those muscles from being harvested and make your body run more efficiently. Eating regularly will also keep your blood-sugar levels constant, which lets your energy and your mood stay elevated.

To gain more muscle and less body fat, it is important to eat less and more often. If you restrict your intake too acutely, the body starts to conserve body fat for fear of starvation on the horizon. It will also conserve energy and slow down the metabolism, so it becomes even harder to lose weight.

DRINK LOTS OF WATER

Your high school health teacher told you this, and it remains good advice: You should consume the equivalent of eight glasses of water a day. The vast majority of our body weight is made up of water, and we need to replenish it regularly. Depriving yourself of water might make you lighter, but it will not help you lose the bad flab. It will instead make it harder for you to get rid of fat.

Dehydration can affect your energy and hunger levels, and it will lower your metabolism by 2–3 percent. That might sound like a small thing, but in the battle against flab, every little bit helps. Water also can be surprisingly satisfying when you are hungry—instead of a candy bar, doughnut, or muffin as a midmorning snack to tide you over until lunch, drink a glass of cold water and you can fight off those hunger pangs.

EAT EIGHT OR MORE SERVINGS OF VEGETABLES AND FRUIT DAILY

Even if you are not a vegetarian, you have to respect the value fruits and veggies offer for a balanced and healthy diet. These foods provide a lot of health benefits, especially those vegetables of darker colors, which contain the most phytochemicals, which are protective chemicals found naturally in plant foods. Vegetables and fruit are typically low in fat and calories, so you will feel satisfied without consuming excess calories. In addition, they contain complex carbohydrates, which are excellent sources of energy.

All vegetables are important, but try to include some good dark green leafy vegetables such as:

- Broccoli

- Collard greens

- Dark leafy lettuce

- Kale

- Mustard greens

- Spinach

Some good, healthy fruits, lower in sugar, are:

- Apples

- Blueberries

- Raspberries

- Strawberries

EAT FISH AND LEGUMES

Red meat contains lots of protein, but you can get similar benefits without as much fat by eating fish and legumes. Alternating between different fish will give you a good and varied protein source—certainly more diverse than a constant stream of fast-food hamburgers. There are many different ways to eat fish: flaked and tossed with salad, grilled, baked. And there are a lot of different flavors to fish. Salmon is hearty, tilapia light, tuna a popular mainstay in many diets. All fish is fine; about three ounces make one helping. Legumes—lentils, chickpeas, black beans, et cetera—are high in protein. About three-quarters of a cup makes one helping.

EAT POULTRY AND EGGS

Most of the fat in a piece of chicken comes from the skin. A three-ounce skinless breast of chicken is low in saturated fat and a good source of protein and iron. Be aware that other cuts of poultry—chicken and turkey—can be high in saturated fat. Eggs eaten whole occasionally are an excellent source of protein; if you eat them regularly, sticking to the egg whites alone is a great way to minimize fat. Try reducing your servings of red meat maybe to three or four times a month during the program. Getting rid of those saturated fats will help you in your battle against flab.

CHOOSE HEALTHY FATS

Fat clogs your arteries, increases your cholesterol, and causes weight gain. But not all fats are created equally. Here are some guidelines.

SATURATED FATS—those that become solid at room temperature, like the fats in butter, fatty dairy products, and lard—are the worst. They are stored that way in the body, too. Limit or avoid such fats and those containing trans-fatty acids. (Trans fats are found in many baked goods as a preservative, and are created when polyunsaturated oils are turned from liquids to solids. There are many health risks associated with trans fats. In 2003, the federal government mandated that food manufacturers label trans-fatty acid content, so pay attention.) These fats contain no nutritional value and are a major culprit in developing heart disease.

UNSATURATED FATS (like vegetable oils) remain liquid at room temperature and are generally better than saturated fats, but there is even a hierarchy there. The "good" fats are those in olive oil (occasionally canola oil), nut butters, nuts, seeds, and avocados—used in moderation, they are a good choice. Even though they are high in fat, it is monounsaturated, which promotes good health. Go easy on polyunsaturated fats found in salad dressings, mayonnaise, and vegetable oils other than olive and canola. The omega-3 fats (also known as linolenic fatty acids) lower triglycerides and cholesterol and are known to lower blood pressure, thereby lowering the risk of heart disease. Flaxseed in any form is an excellent source of omega-3 fat.

EXCESS FAT is stored under the skin as body fat. You can eat the same number of grams of carbohydrates and protein as fat and take in fewer calories, which requires you to work less to lose weight. You can eat plates of vegetables before racking up the same number of unwanted calories as are found in a handful of potato chips, which are high in fat.

EAT WHOLE GRAINS

Whole grains, especially in the form of brown rice, quinoa, and oatmeal, are good for the body. Grains provide the complex carbohydrates the body needs to keep blood-sugar levels balanced. Eating whole-grain breads occasionally—say, once a day—is also an acceptable source of carbs. But beware of refined carbs such as those found in white breads, white rice, and pasta. These can cause a surge in blood-sugar levels, resulting in low energy. They tend to be metabolized as sugar and therefore lead to weight gain.

EAT THREE HIGH-CALCIUM FOODS A DAY

Calcium strengthens bones and enriches the cells of the body. It serves a vital role in bone structure, providing density and integrity to your skeleton.

One cup of calcium and vitamin D–fortified soy milk is an ideal source, as are one ounce of soy cheese, four ounces of tofu (145 milligrams of calcium), three ounces of fish (sardines have a whopping 372 milligrams of calcium), and a serving of dark green leafy vegetables. (Surprisingly, these veggies are relatively high in calcium.) If you eat dairy, try one cup of low-fat milk, one ounce of cheese, or one cup of plain low-fat yogurt (one of the highest sources of calcium—415 milligrams). The daily amount the body requires varies with size and age, but 1,000 milligrams of calcium per day is a good target.

DANGER ZONES (AND HOW TO AVOID THEM)

The nemesis of healthy eating is lazy eating. Even people who are active and don't think they eat too much may be surprised to find that they never seem to lose weight. That might not be because they are overeating, but because they are *incorrectly* eating.

Remember what we learned earlier: The body burns off foods in a particular order: sugars first, complex carbohydrates second, fats last. If you eat a lot of fatty foods, you store that fat on your body and decrease the effectiveness of exercise because you are always adding fat to your diet, and you will have to work twice as hard to get rid of it.

But the same is true if you consume excessive amounts of sugar. Imagine that your diet were nothing but sugars. Because sugar is first in line, you would always be burning off the first layer of fuel, never getting toward your reserves of fat. Remember, you have two levels of fuel to expel before you make the flab drop off, and lots of sugar keeps you always in the first and second layer, never the third. Sugars, in short, are empty calories that are not your friend!

You need to know something about body chemistry to understand that even items that do not appear to have sugar in them can be bad for you. Alcohol, for example, does not contain sugar, but it is converted to it in the body. It also primes your cells to store more fat. Best not to drink too much, and save the bubbly and beer for that special occasion only.

The best way to avoid the dangers of poor food choices is to be aware of what you put into your body. Fried foods are high in fats because they are cooked in oil. If you are going to consume fried foods, try to prepare them in olive or canola oil, and use only as much as you need. Allow the food to drain as thoroughly as possible before eating. You are better off baking your foods, which is generally much healthier—and grilling is even better!

Fast food is full of hidden calories, and because you never see it being prepared, you really don't know all that goes into it. Cooking at home is not only cheaper, it's also a lot better for you.

Be aware of what you are taking in and how much; then control the bad and increase the good. This, combined with my exercise program, will result in improvements in your appearance and how you feel that will simply amaze you.

CHAPTER 4

The Role of Emotions in Fighting Flab

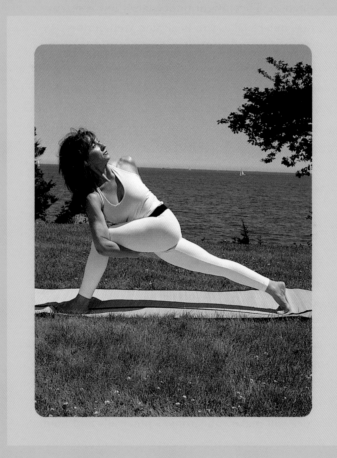

A positive emotional approach lets us do more than just survive—it gives us a healthy outlook toward living our lives. Being positive and optimistic is a key element in achieving a healthy body as well. Instead of focusing on the things that make us unhappy, we concentrate on the good and expand from there. This infiltrates all aspects of our lives.

Some people are skeptical of the benefits of yoga, especially the aspect that embraces meditation. They might understand how resistance training increases muscles, but not how quiet makes you healthier. Well, it does. As *Time* magazine reported in an August 2003 cover story, "Not only do studies show that meditation is boosting [practitioners'] immune systems, but brain scans suggest that it may be rewiring their brains to reduce stress … Meditation is being recommended by more and more physicians as a way to prevent, slow or at least control the pain of chronic diseases like heart conditions, AIDS, cancer and infertility … Scientific studies are beginning to show it works, particularly for stress-related conditions." In short, even Western doctors acknowledge that meditation, a key aspect of yoga, leads to better physical health, not just mental acuity.

A HEALTHY MIND MEANS A HEALTHY FLAB-FREE BODY

A healthy mind dictates optimism and elevates your emotional well-being. Focusing on the upside will also make you healthier, mentally and physically, because you want to enjoy life and want to feel healthy and strong through exercise and living a healthier lifestyle. Pessimism lowers your immunity and detracts from your focus on exercising regularly and eating sensibly. Yoga is like a gift for your mind. The rewards of a frequent yoga practice are almost immediate—you will notice increased mental clarity, efficiency, and self-confidence. Your practice will show you what peace of mind really feels like.

Your practice will make you stronger physically and mentally. You will gain confidence as you discover new postures, focus your mind and energy, feel the power of your control, and see the weight slipping away as you reshape your mind and body.

STRESS AND ITS ASSOCIATION WITH FLAB

Stress from too much pressure and/or aggravation has many negative effects on our mental and physical health. Chronic stress can lead to long-term ill health. Stress hormones such as cortisol are released, turning on fat-cell storage throughout the body, especially in the abdomen.

We do live in a stressful society, and it is hard to avoid stress, but we can use tools to deal with it. Rather than exploding from the pressures of day-to-day living, you can use yoga as your stress-release button. Yoga is widely known as one of the best tools for releasing tension—a powerful yoga session followed by deep relaxation brings a wonderful gift of peacefulness to your body and spirit, banishing stress.

The main cause of stress is an overactive mind—we obsess over things we cannot control, think too much about the negative, worry over the future. The way yoga helps you de-stress is by slowing you down on the inside. This will immediately reduce stress, and help you live life deliberately and unhurriedly. It also helps us slow down on the outside. When we get overly busy, we slip out of good behavior and back into our old addictive habits. This means we might overeat and skip workouts, which contribute to more flab and less good health.

YOUR BODY IMAGE

One of the great benefits of your practice of yoga is how it helps build a positive view of your body. I can practically guarantee that you will gain more compassion toward yourself within the first week of poses. Your true inner nature is lifted by the discipline and freedom of the postures, and you can see and become more in tune with yourself. You will gain respect and admiration for yourself and for Mother Nature, gaining a non-judgmental attitude.

The yoga practices outlined in the book will also help you burn fat, which will surely make you feel better about yourself—and others will see you more positively, too. People who are physically active are perceived as hardworking, more self-confident and self-disciplined, and more sexually attractive compared to those who do not exercise. Activity gives your skin a healthy glow and you radiate happiness.

As you begin, take a realistic look at yourself. It is very important to be realistic when starting on any body-fat reduction program. There are certain factors that are hereditary and that we cannot really control, characteristics we cannot truly change: our height, the length of our legs, our skin tone, and the color of our hair. (Of course, we can give the appearance of changing these things with high-heel shoes, tanning booths, and hair dye, but the truth of them is always within our bodies.)

Unfortunately, certain aspects of our body types are hard to change, as they have been passed down to us in our genes. As I said earlier, every body is different and requires its own proportion of body fat. A slow metabolism means some people simply do not burn flab as efficiently as others do. Moreover, as our bodies grow and develop, many attributes of our own past abandon us—our bodies do slow down and process foods and activities differently.

Nevertheless, there are some results of heredity that we do have some control over. It is amazing what a substantial and dramatic change lessening the body fat can make in our overall health. Toning, sculpting, and losing body fat can make you appear taller, slimmer, and stronger than your genes have allowed for. Defined muscles and a relatively low level of body fat are the flab-fighting secret!

But you must always be realistic about what you can achieve with what you have to work with. Think of Arnold Schwarzenegger and Brad Pitt. Both are extremely fit, handsome specimens. But no matter how hard he works out, Brad will probably never look like Arnold—his body type is different, his frame is different, his positive traits are his own. You cannot change the essence of who you are, and you should not want to. You can only get fit and allow your inner light to shine through and make you the best you you can be!

BE CLEAR ON YOUR GOALS

If you are practicing yoga to fight flab, keep that goal in mind and remember not to allow yourself to become impatient with the pace or angry with yourself if it takes a little longer to achieve your goals. When you practice with a specific goal in mind, your practice is more productive, directed, and beneficial in every way.

POSITIVE THINKING, MEDITATION, AND VISUALIZATION

Some happy tone
Of meditation, slipping in between
The beauty coming and the beauty gone.

        ≈ WILLIAM WORDSWORTH, *Most Sweet It Is* (1835)

You will plug into positive thinking as a result of practicing your yoga sessions—you will develop a soft and subtle strength from your asanas (poses) as you get strong and healthy, mentally and physically.

This is not simply Eastern mysticism masquerading as science. Dr. Mehmet Oz, a cardiovascular surgeon at New York's Columbia Presbyterian Medical Center, has written about how he prescribes meditation and yoga to prepare patients for surgery because, he says simply, "it works."

Meditation is the active process of encouraging stillness in the mind. When practicing meditation we withdraw the mind from the onslaught of daily pressures and tune into an inner oasis of calm—even just a few minutes of meditation each day can drastically improve our ability to cope with everyday life and help us develop an awareness of inner calm.

Meditation is at the heart of every style of yoga. Through meditation, yoga affects not only the body, but also the mind. Through meditation, you will experience peace, calm, and a greater sense of focus. There are many ways to meditate during this program.

Many of my students find that they are better able to meditate in their postures while moving—they find that sitting still and trying to erase thoughts is counterproductive and ineffective. So try it. You may need to approach your meditation practice in different ways to find one that suits you best. When you happen upon it, stick with it.

Once your yoga advances, the poses and practices will become their own kind of meditation. I have been a fan of yoga for only eight years, and I found early on that yoga made me so focused, put me so in the moment, that I meditate not only throughout my personal sessions, but also throughout the classes I teach. This ability came with time. Narrowing the gaps between your thoughts and stilling your mind is the essence of meditation.

By getting in touch with your core, your breath, and by staying in the moment while practicing the postures, you will begin to meditate. This will happen subtly, as you progress in your regimen. Be aware that it is happening, and enjoy it for the wonder that it will bring to your life.

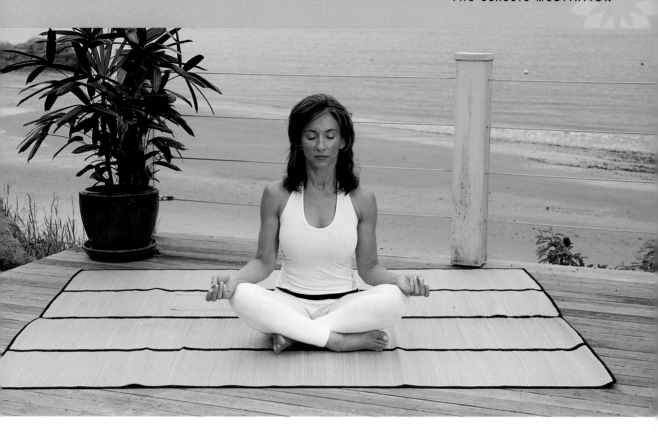

The Classic Meditation

DIRECTIONS

1. Sit on the floor, crossed-leg position. Rest your hands on your knees. Relax your shoulders.

2. Start breathing consciously.

3. As you inhale, imagine you are drawing in positive energy for achieving your confidence goals, for your success and accomplishments, for your patience and for your laughter.

4. As you exhale, imagine you are breathing out all the negative energy, the feelings of fear, failure, impatience, or sadness.

5. Continue to observe the breath, inhaling positive thoughts and actualizing them, exhaling all the negative thoughts associated with a self-limiting mind-set.

6. Repeat for 10 to 20 breaths.

7. Continue by lying down and getting into the Corpse pose for the next 5 to 10 minutes in deep silence.

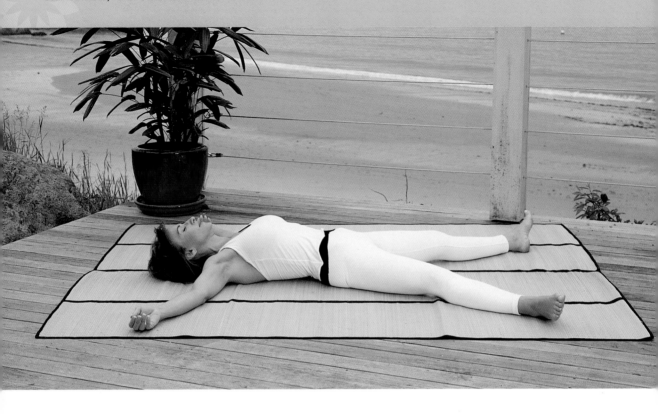

Savasana, or Corpse Pose

DIRECTIONS

1 Lie flat on your back with your feet apart and your toes relaxed and facing out.

2 Place your arms out from your sides, with your palms up.

3 Close your eyes and consciously release and relax each and every muscle, transferring all the weight of your body to the floor.

4 Slowly bring your focus to your breath, and feel the rhythmic movement of your body as you breathe in and out. Really get in touch with your body and your breath, holding the pose for 5 to 10 minutes.

5 Wrap your arms around your knees, drawing them into your chest, and roll to your right side into a fetal position.

VISUALIZATION TECHNIQUES

Positive visualization is a powerful tool for yoga students. Thinking positive thoughts and visualizing yourself accomplishing your goals are important steps toward finding peace and the resolve to change your life.

Yoga will help you create a healthy self-image. Give yourself time at the end of each session to release negative thoughts and replace them with positive thoughts. Focus by using your exhalation to release tired and old self-limiting thoughts, and your inhalation to bring on the new and positive thoughts.

- ☞ FOCUS ON YOUR BREATH. From the beginning, focus or concentrate on your breath, because the breath is the essence of meditation. A useful technique is to count your breaths during each pose, counting forward and backward, focusing your attention on what you are doing. Slow your breath with deep, long inhalations and exhalations. Stay with this technique throughout your session. This is the essence of meditation on breath.

- ☞ FOCUS ON YOUR POSTURES. You can meditate during your practice by placing your total focus on the postures you are performing. Get in the moment and stay there. Focus on where you're placing your hand, your foot. Pay attention to how it feels to twist your spine, and feel your body's reaction to the challenging postures and stretches. Focus all your attention on what you are doing. This is meditation in motion.

- ☞ FOCUS ON GAZING. Gazing at an image during your yoga session can serve as a successful portal in meditation. Think of something blissful and keep focusing on it in your mind. Whether it's a candle's flame or a loved one's face, keep it in the front of your mind and bring your attention back to it as you come into and go out of the poses. You can also focus on something tangible in the room, like a spot on the floor or an item on the wall. It will amaze you how focusing visually on an object brings balance to the body and to the mind. It's proof that the eye, and therefore the mind, controls the body.

FOCUS ON VISUALIZATION. Meditate during your session by visualizing yourself on a beautiful beach or in another natural place, experiencing the waves of the ocean, looking at the blue sky, hearing the sounds of nature. A CD of appropriate music can help you focus on your vision. It will give your mind a focal point and help you to still the chatter in your head.

Concentrate on *positive* thoughts while inhaling; concentrate on *negative* thoughts while exhaling.

INHALE	EXHALE
Self-confidence	*Self-doubt*
Accomplishment	*Fear*
Success	*Failure*
Patience	*Impatience*
Laughter	*Sadness*

FIVE FLAB-FIGHTING BENEFITS OF MEDITATION

Let's be frank—all the meditation in the world will not help you lose weight if you do not get your body moving and eat fewer calories than you use. But there are undeniable benefits that meditation affords in setting your goals and finding the discipline to achieve them. Meditation alone does not burn fat—it makes your body's ability to rid itself of fat faster possible! Here are five tangible benefits of meditation.

1. DECREASES MENTAL STRESS AND BODY TENSION. *Stress robs us of concentration and leads us toward unproductive activities, whether snacking or getting distracted from our exercise routine. Tension burns nothing but years off your life. Establishing control over these negative energies enables you to direct more attention toward positive energies.*

2. **LEAVES YOU FEELING REFRESHED, REJUVENATED, AND OPTIMISTIC.** *Every parent knows that allowing a child to nap for just a short while in the middle of the day lets that child go on to the evening. Think of meditation as a kind of adult nap that frees the mind and gives you the energy to attack your day with more gusto! Activity reduces flab, and meditation expands your ability to engage in that activity.*

3. **DECREASES BLOOD PRESSURE.** *The dangers of high blood pressure are obvious. The heart can fail due to overwork. Meditation relaxes the body and mind, promoting overall health. Some of my clients with high blood pressure have told me that after several months of practicing yoga, their doctors have reduced their medication. The reason is that yoga asanas, or postures, help you bring your mind to stillness. You will quiet your mind because these poses take a lot of mental concentration, and as a result, you stay in the moment with no thought ... this is meditation. So, you are, in essence, practicing meditation with your yoga postures.*

4. **SLOWS DOWN BRAIN ACTIVITY AND BRINGS CLARITY.** *Meditation helps you bring your mind to a place of stillness. By quieting our minds, we slow down our brain activity and remove clutter, which creates a positive mental balance. Withdrawing your attention from outside objects and concerns will concentrate energies internally and promote inner health.*

5. **FOCUSES THE MIND AND AIDS IN VISUALIZATION.** *A good attitude empowers us to achieve things we might have thought were outside of our grasp. If you can visualize your ability to do something, you are better prepared to achieve that goal.*

During your meditation or your yoga session, visualize how you would like to see yourself, tuning in to all the positive aspects of your image.

CHAPTER 5

The Total 30-Day Flab-Burning Program

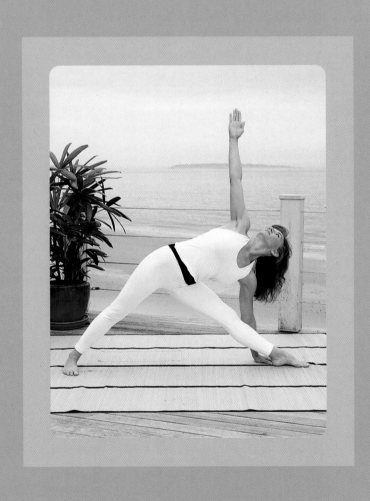

Now that we all understand the mechanics of our workout and the importance of sensible eating, we can get ready to begin the actual Total 30-Day Flab-Burning Program.

This is a program of my own design that has been geared toward reducing flab on any number of body types.

The harder your muscles have to work, the more calories you burn—flab loss is reducing calories in and increasing calories out—so let's start burning up those calories!

☞ As with any exercise regimen, check with your doctor before you begin to ensure that using this at-home program of self-supervised exercises is right for you, and that you are not at risk for any injuries.

☞ If you have not exercised for a long time, take things slowly and build up in increments. The program is designed for anyone from novice to expert, with certain challenges inserted to increase the demands of the workout.

☞ You should not feel totally exhausted after a yoga workout, but rather stretched and refreshed. If you do feel exhausted, tone it down a little. The beauty of yoga is the overall feeling of well-being it promotes without doing violence to your systems.

☞ Remember the magic three—that means, by the third day you will become even more enthusiastic, your practice will flow that much easier, and you will welcome the challenge of doing more, not less.

OVERVIEW OF THE PROGRAM

My program comprises seven different challenging yoga sessions for each day of the week. Each day includes a cardiovascular routine for direct body-fat burning, and an anaerobic yoga session where we use muscle-strengthening postures coupled with stretching. Remember, increased muscle strength means more flab-burning—for maximum results!

Every day is designed to focus on one particular style of pose that targets a different area of the body or technique for promoting a trimmer you. Day One is comprised of Standing Strengthening Poses; Day Two is devoted to Balancing Poses; Day Three to Twisting Poses; Day Four to Back Strengthening Poses; Day Five to Abdominal Strengthening Poses; Day Six to Sculpting and Toning Upper Body Poses; Day Seven to Lower Body Sculpting Poses. Days Eight through Thirty refine and increase the challenge level to these poses, until you are a fat-burning engine.

You really need to commit to the program for the first month to give you a real boost and reveal the new you. The twenty-four hours between each session will be sufficient to allow your muscles to recover, but I have programmed in two rest days. If you do miss a day, don't be hard on yourself—just continue the day after that. If you are ill, really listen to your body. If you have a really heavy cold, flu, or fever, you won't feel like exercising … so don't do it! Give your body a few days to feel better and fight off the infection. It is important to keep up with the program, but taking a few days off every now and then will not impair the overall results. The most important advice I can give you is to listen to your body.

WEEK ONE

Every day must begin with a warm-up to set the stage for your exercise. There are two different warm-up routines herein, which you can alternate to keep your program fresh. (See pages 51 and 60.) Following your warm-up, engage in the cardiovascular training. The Super-Efficient Walk or Walk/Run Workout will get your heart pumping. (See page 66.)

Proceed on a daily basis, starting with Day One and continuing through Day Seven. (See pages 94 through 160.)

Finish each day with cooldowns for upper and lower body. There are two of each in the book, to be used alternately—one upper-body cooldown and one lower-body cooldown every day. (See pages 68 and 76 for lower-body, and pages 80 and 84 for upper-body.) End every routine with Savasana—the resting period. (See page 40.)

WEEK TWO THROUGH WEEK FOUR

We'll get into more detail later on, but the subsequent weeks are meant to build upon the lessons you've already learned, and increase in the degree of challenge.

You'll repeat the warm-ups, cardio, cooldowns, and Savasana as well as the routines from Day One to Day Seven. Take note that while the general routines are the same, to give you a sense of continuity, the instructions for subsequent weeks (at the end of the chapter) increase difficulty with challenge poses and include two built-in rest days. (See pages 162-163.)

BEYOND WEEK FOUR

After you have made the routines a habit for thirty days, you will find yourself so energized and refreshed that you might want to do the poses every day after that. If you do, I say, congratulations! I practice yoga virtually every day because I love it; I know you will love it, too, but not everyone can devote every day to the exercises. You can achieve valuable maintenance practicing yoga only three or four times a week. Imagine: A flab-free body and healthy mind for the rest of your life, and it only takes two hours a week in the privacy of your own home!

Devise a maintenance regimen that works for you. As long as you spend just thirty minutes a day, three or fours days a week, practicing your postures, you will not only remain fit and feel great, but you will keep the flab off. I suggest trying one of these maintenance programs:

1. *Practice the exercises from Day One to Day Seven—some weeks you'll do three days, some weeks, four.*

2. *If you wish to practice four times a week, do the poses for Day One to Day Four one week, then those for Day Four to Day Seven the next.*

3. *Whenever you wish to challenge yourself, go back to practicing every day.*

By practicing each week, you will improve your body's ability to replace fat with muscle and melt away unwanted flab. Take each day step-by-step, and the results will be totally amazing!

Each day will present you with different challenges. These are designed to take you to higher levels of achievement. And though each day is challenging in its own way, taken together, this program will form the complete flab-fighting workout! Adding additional challenges is something you can do at your own discretion. If you find yourself not ready to meet the challenges I present on the days I present them, don't despair! You can always add more breaths or more repetitions when you are ready.

Always listen to your body. It will tell you how fast to proceed. Every individual's body is different and each person's level of fitness or lack of fitness is different. Go at the pace that is comfortable for you. You will grow in increments and you will reach your goal!

BEFORE YOU BEGIN

ENVIRONMENT

Proper yoga practice requires an environment conducive to cleansing the body. The room you practice in should not go below 78 degrees so your muscles stay warm. Wear workout gear that is comfortable. Feel free to add relaxing music to your exercise in order to soothe the mind and promote meditation along with the exercises.

WARMING UP

A warm-up is exactly what it sounds like—a way of creating heat within the body and gradually speeding up the circulation of your whole body, through balanced stretches and counterstretches. Building heat in the body will build up heat in the muscles, making them more pliable and less prone to tearing or pulling injuries. It is crucial to warm up every time you exercise—it ensures that you begin and end your program safely.

COOLING DOWN

Equally important as the warm-up is what comes *after* your yoga workout. A good cooling down will leave you refreshed and invigorated by your workout and not exhausted. Stopping any exercise suddenly when your heart and blood are pumping vigorously could cause a blockage—the circulatory system needs time to return to a more normal pace. Muscles also need to be released from strong contractions with adequate stretching.

Many students I see in my classes live life in the fast lane and leave before the cooldown—you may have to force yourself to take the time for relaxation exercises at the end of your workout, including Savasana. Just remember, operating at full power means you need to recharge your batteries!

STRETCHING

Stretching is a major part of the warm-ups and cooldowns. Stretching takes only a few minutes and is invaluable. It will minimize your risk of injuries, your muscles will feel less sore, and your flexibility will increase.

BREATHING

Princes and lords may flourish, or may fade;
A breach can make them, as a breath has made …

　OLIVER GOLDSMITH, *Edwin and Angelina, or the Hermit* (1764)

Most people do not understand the importance of breathing correctly. More so even than water, breath is the source of vital life force. We can go days without a drop of water, but only minutes without taking a breath. Yet few exercise regimens give breathing the attention it is due for its importance in overall good health.

When you exercise control over your breathing, you can learn to control the subtle energies within your body, and as a result gain full control over the mind. Yoga teaches proper breathing techniques that can help you unite your body and mind.

Part of your yoga program should be mastering what I call the Complete Breath. But even when you are not practicing particular poses, the Complete Breath is something you can add to your daily life—you can do it when you get up in the morning, when you are riding up to the office in the elevator, when you are sitting at a traffic light. The more full and thorough introduction of oxygen into your lungs benefits your entire body as the oxygen passes through it, refreshing the muscles and purifying the blood. Your body will work more efficiently and therefore burn flab faster!

THE COMPLETE BREATH

This is a full, deep, and slow breath. Be conscious of fully using the lungs. You need to increase lung capacity, which will efficiently cleanse the blood.

DIRECTIONS:

1. *Exhale, clearing the lungs before you begin.*

2. *Inhale, filling up the bottom of your lungs, the middle of your lungs, then slowly filling the chest. Feel your abdomen rise, then your diaphragm, and finally your chest.*

3. *Exhale, slowly emptying the lungs from the top to the bottom.*

4. *For optimum health, breathing should be long, deep, full, and rhythmic—it should completely fill and empty your lungs. Short, rapid breathing and holding your breath deprive your body of oxygen.*

When practicing yoga poses, remember to keep your abdominal muscles firm and slightly contracted. Breathe in an unbroken rhythm through your nose, keeping your mouth closed.

WARM-UPS

Here are two different warm-up routines. You should alternate between them in your daily regimen—do Warm-up One on even-numbered days, Warm-up Two on odd-numbered, or whatever system works for you. The variety is intended to give you good results while keeping the program fresh and lively.

Warm-up One

Practice these eight postures fairly quickly to prepare yourself, moving on to Warm-up Two on alternate days.

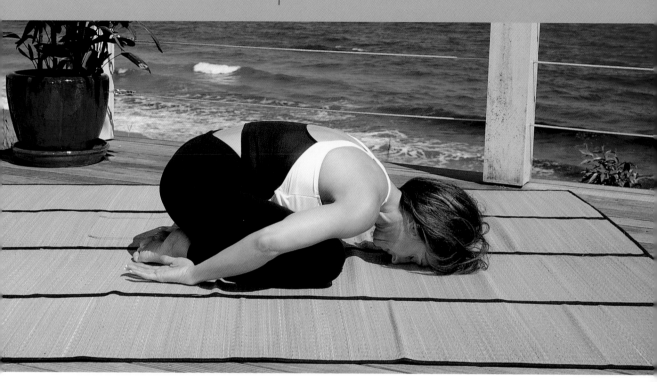

Child's Pose

STRETCHES: *Spine and thigh muscles*

IMPROVES: *Circulation*

The Child's Pose reduces fatigue and tension and relaxes your lower back and neck. It slows down the heart rate and calms emotions.

DIRECTIONS

1. Kneel on the floor and bring your buttocks toward your heels.

2. Place your arms lengthwise alongside your body.

3. Stretch your chin forward to the floor, rounding your spine and shoulders.

4. Relax your neck muscles and relax into the pose. Hold this pose for 3 breaths.

Cat's Pose

STRENGTHENS AND TONES: *Upper back*
STRETCHES: *Spine*
IMPROVES: *Flexibility*

This pose opens the spine and releases tension in the muscles of the neck and shoulders. This pose is particularly effective for stretching and opening the spine, shoulders, and neck and for counteracting the effects of poor posture.

DIRECTIONS

1. Get on all fours, with your palms flat on the floor directly below your shoulders and your knees directly below your hips.

2. Inhale while contracting your abdominal muscles. Round your back, dropping your head toward the floor.

3. Exhale while releasing your abdominal muscles, arching your spine, lifting your head, and sticking your buttocks out and up. All of the arching and rounding of your spine should initiate from your pelvis.

4. Repeat the pose 3 times.

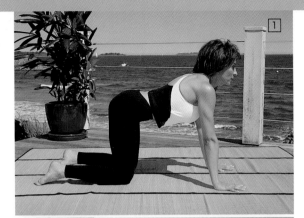

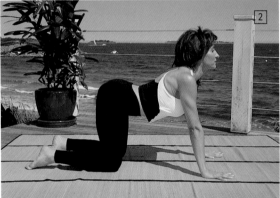

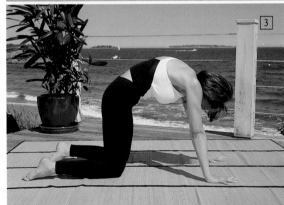

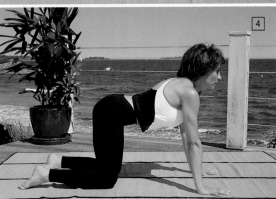

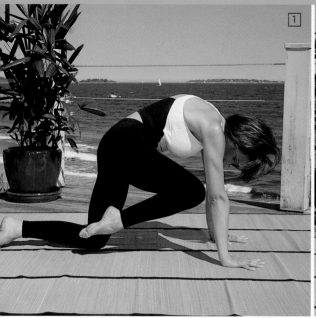

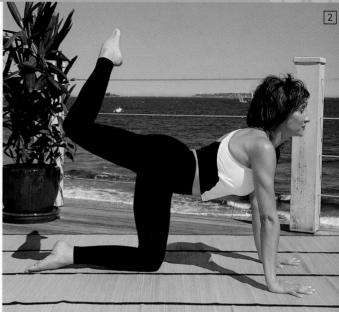

Cat's Pose Extended

STRENGTHENS AND TONES: *Upper back, Abdominals*

STRETCHES: *Spine*

IMPROVES: *Flexibility*

This pose strengthens and tones the hamstrings and buttocks and the muscles of the back and abs.

DIRECTIONS

1. From the Cat's Pose on all fours, inhale while contracting your abdominal muscles, rounding your back and bringing in your knee toward your forehead.

2. Exhale while releasing your abdominal muscles, arching your spine, lifting your head, and extending your right leg back behind you toward the sky.

3. Repeat 3 times.

4. Repeat with your left leg.

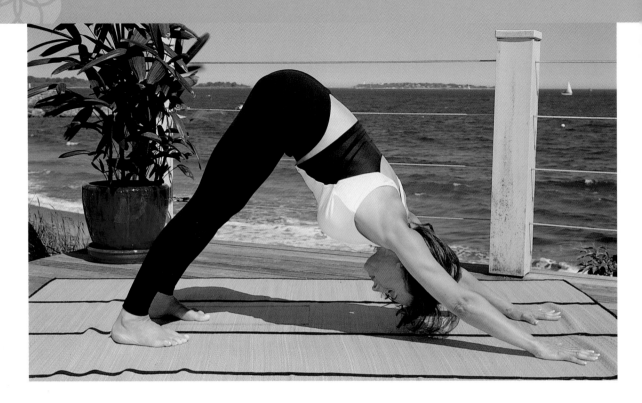

Downward Facing Dog

STRENGTHENS AND TONES: *Arms*
STRETCHES: *Back, Hips, Shoulders*
IMPROVES: *Circulation to the head and face*

If you have a dog, you have no doubt marveled at his flexibility—and supreme sense of refreshment and relaxation—when he awakes from a nap curled up on your ottoman. That is the essence of this pose, which stretches from the hips to the neck and the whole back side of the body.

DIRECTIONS

1 From the Cat's Pose, straighten your legs and shift your weight toward your heels and hips. Reach your arms as far forward as you can, and keep your hands and feet shoulder-width apart.

2 Fan out your fingers, making sure to keep your palms pressed evenly on the floor.

3 Lift your tailbone upward, keeping your knees bent as necessary.

4 Shift your weight back toward your hips and pull your shoulder blades back toward your waist. Your weight should be evenly distributed between your hands and feet.

5 Drop your head toward the floor and deliberately release your neck muscles. Hold this pose for 5 breaths.

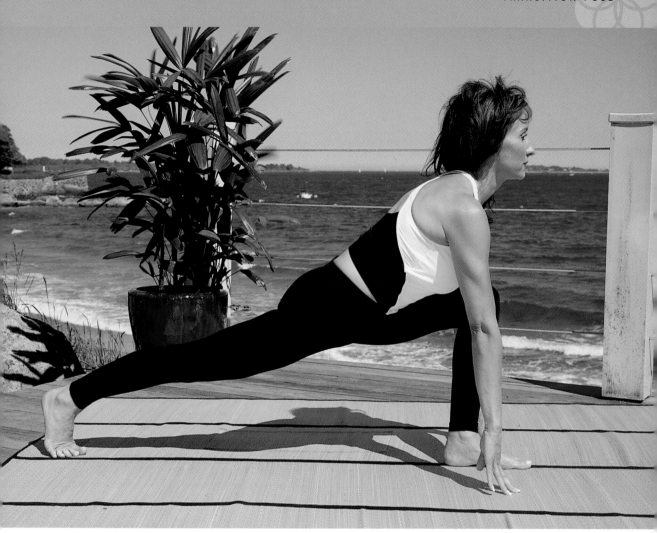

Transition Pose

DIRECTIONS

1. From the Downward Facing Dog, bring your left foot between your hands, then your right foot. Raise your torso.

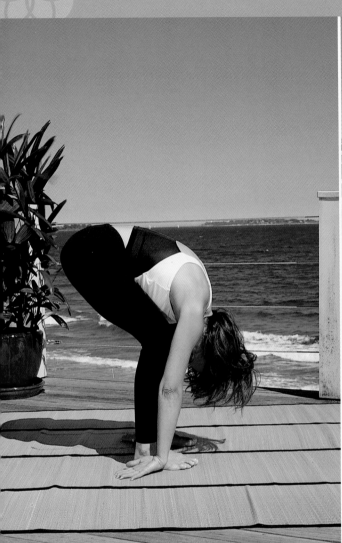
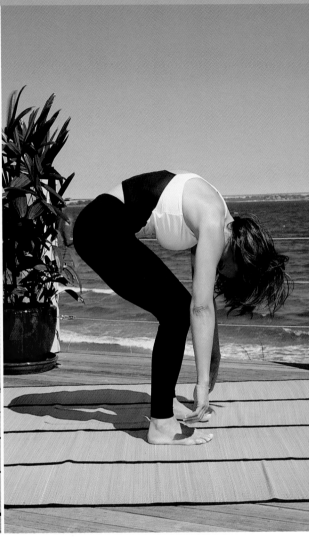

Rag Doll Roll-up

DIRECTIONS

1 From the Transition Pose, bring both feet together, slowly roll your body and relax the back of your neck. Let the weight of your head pull your neck, making it long, while you roll your body to a standing position.

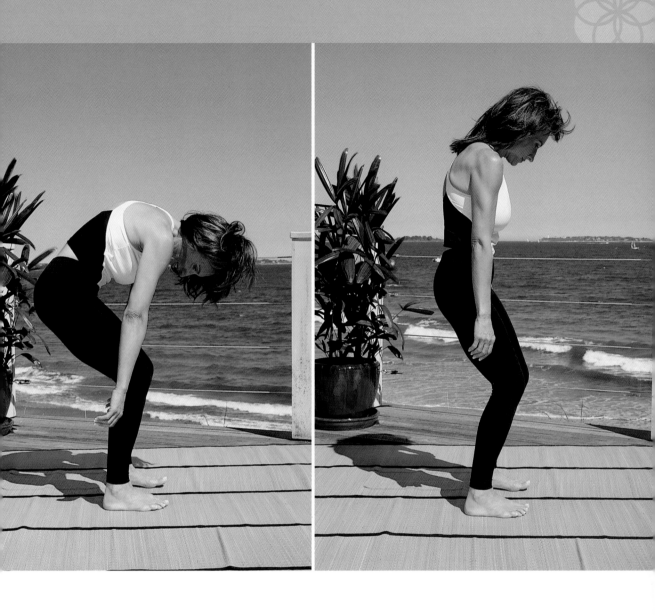

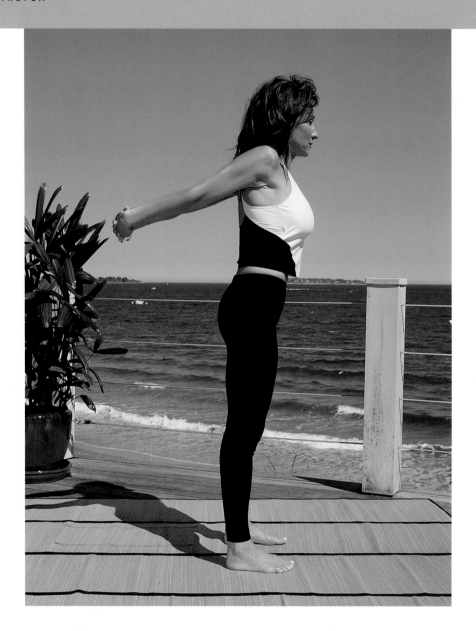

Back Stretch

DIRECTIONS

1   Interlace your fingers behind your back and lift your arms as high as you can.

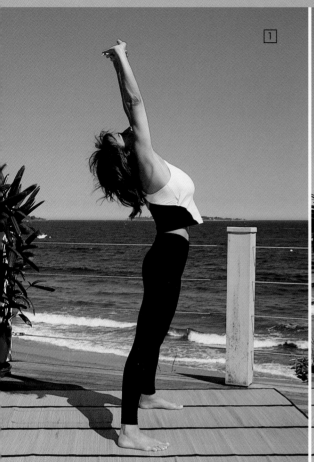

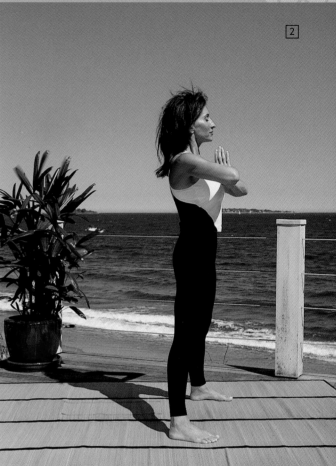

Full Length Stretch

DIRECTIONS

1 From a standing position, interlace your fingers. Stretch your arms all the way over your head and gently release your head, letting it fall back. Feel the stretch from your waist all the way up to your hands.

2 Bring your hands together to your heart center and close your eyes. Take 2 long, deep breaths, inhaling and exhaling completely. Feel yourself reaching down to the bottom of your lungs.

Warm-up Two

1 2   3 4

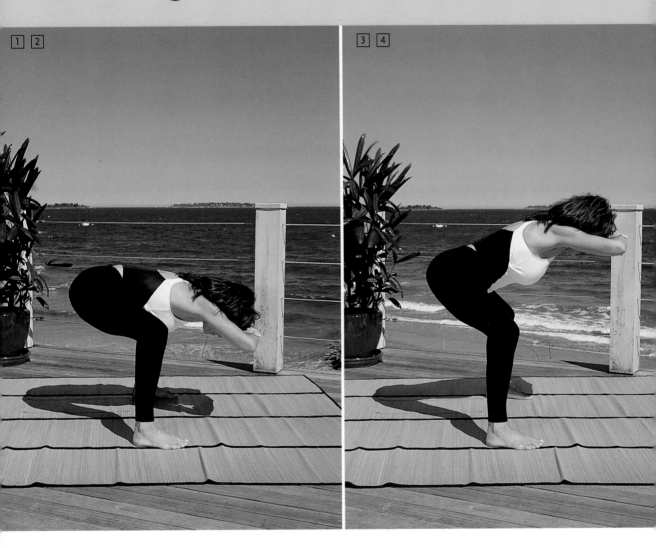

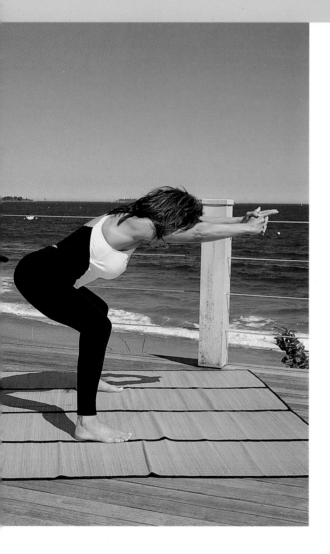

Moving Forward Bend—Knees Bent

IMPROVES: *Overall flexibility*

This will start to awaken your spine and your body.

DIRECTIONS

1. From a standing position, bend your knees.

2. Fold your body forward, holding your elbows.

3. Inhale, lifting your arms (while still holding your elbows) a little higher.

4. Exhale, lowering your elbows a little lower and awakening the spine.

5. Still with bent knees, extend your arms forward.

> *continued on next page*

6 Extend arms to your sides, and then back behind you, interlacing your fingers.

7 Raise your arms behind you as high as you can.

8 Straighten your legs and lift your arms even higher to get a good stretch. Come back to standing position.

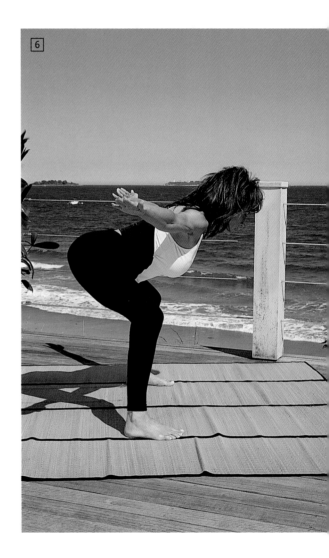

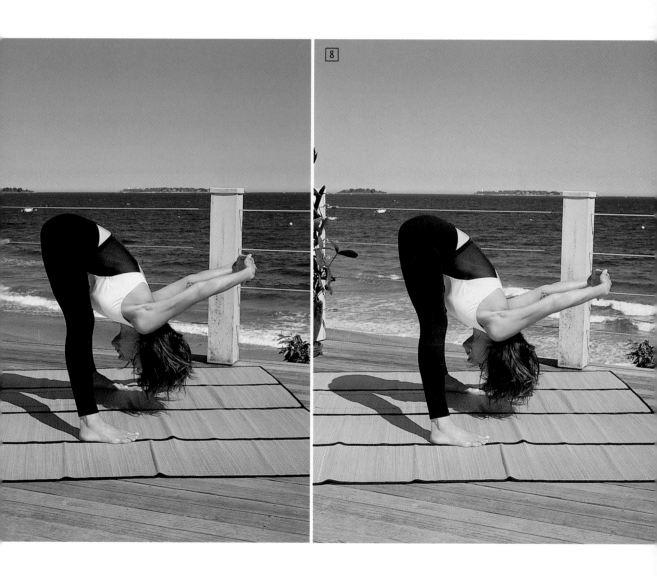

8

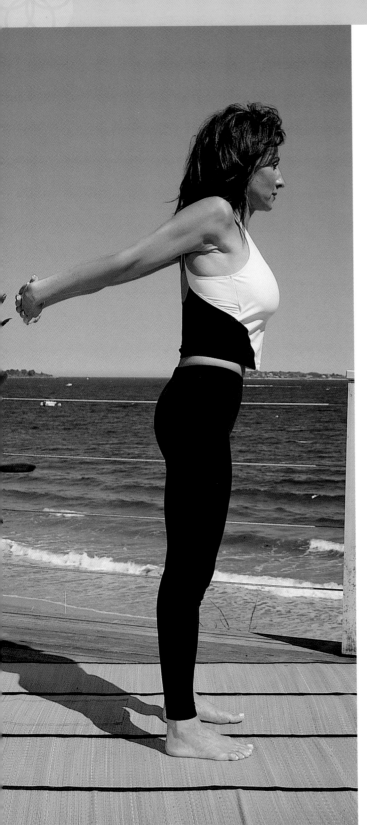

Back Stretch

STRETCHES: *Arms, Neck, Shoulders*

IMPROVES: *Flexibility*

This pose will increase flexibility and release tension and stiffness in your arms and neck.

DIRECTIONS

1. Keeping your fingers interlaced behind your back, lift your arms as high as you can.

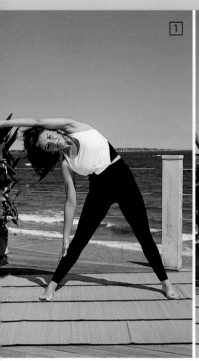
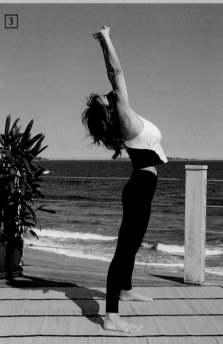
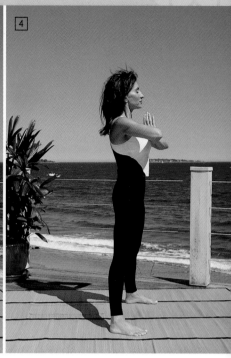

Lateral Side Stretch and Full Length Stretch

IMPROVES: *Flexibility*

This pose increases flexibility to your spine and the sides of the waist. It will also loosen your leg and hip muscles.

DIRECTIONS

1. While standing straight up, unclasp your hands and stretch your left arm all the way over to the right, getting a nice lateral stretch to the waist.

2. Slowly return your body to a straight standing position. Switch arms and stretch your right arm all the way over to the left for a stretch to the other side of the waist.

3. Slowly return your body to the straight standing position. Interlace your fingers and stretch your arms all the way over your head. Gently release your head, letting it fall back. Feel the stretch from your waist all the way up to your pointed fingers.

4. Bring your hands to your heart center and close your eyes. Take 2 long, deep breaths, inhaling and exhaling completely. Feel yourself reaching down to the bottom of your lungs.

Cardio Training

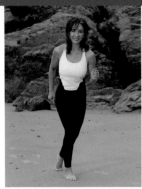 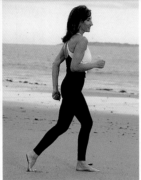

The Super-Efficient Walk or Walk/Run Workout

As a fitness trainer, yoga advisor, and teacher, I come across many runners, novice and professional. Long-term running or jogging can be very hard on the joints, especially the knees, and tightening to the hamstrings. Adding a walking element decreases the intensity of running by itself. In this way, you will get an equally demanding workout. Brisk walking is just as efficient as the walk/run—it's mostly a personal choice—but either way, you will burn significant calories and boost your heart rate. This cardio program will increase your metabolism and help blast away the fat.

DIRECTIONS

1 Find somewhere you can do a continuous walk with a minimum of roadblocks and interruptions such as traffic. Out in the open with nature is the best choice; barring that, a shopping mall, empty parking lot, or quiet park or walking trail will do. Set your watch and walk continually for 15 minutes at a brisk pace.

2 As a bonus burner, walk so fast that you break into a run intermittently. When you are walking for fitness you should be breathing fairly heavily—don't dawdle! Walk purposefully.

3 The most important technique to master for proper brisk walking or running is breathing. The proper breath is a very deep inhalation and exhalation. People who tend to take rapid, shallow breaths create carbon-dioxide buildup in their cells, increase their heart rate, and encourage muscle cramps. Deep breaths get more oxygen to your muscles, rid your body of carbon dioxide, and aid in reducing fatigue. If your upper body, fists, or face is clenched while running, the blood that should be going to your legs is sent to the flexed or tensed body parts as well, and this will decrease the amount of oxygen to your legs. Relax and breathe deeply.

The Stairs Climb Workout

DIRECTIONS:

1   Use your stairs at home or some steps at the beach or local park for 15 minutes of cardiovascular work.

2   Walk/run up and down the stairs.

3   Walk/run up and down the stairs two at a time. Watch your technique—your knees should be in line with your toes as you step upward, and on the way down, pull in your abdominal muscles to support your back and step through your toes to the heel to protect your knees while stepping down at a slant. Your breathing should be deep and slow, not shallow.

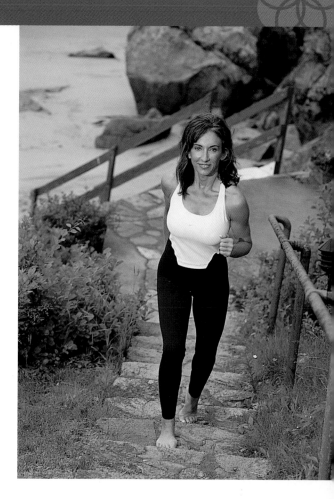

The Walk/Run and Stairs Climb cardio routines are big-time flab fighters that burn significant calories while sending your spirits soaring. The treadmill is okay, but the beauty of this cardio program is that all you need is a good pair of shoes and nature—somewhere to walk and run. This will build cardiovascular endurance, get your heart rate up, and set the calorie- and fat-burning process in motion.

Cooldown Stretches

Once again, alternate between the two lower-body stretches and the two upper-body stretches, as you like. The important thing is not to skip this vital step. It allows your body to cool down, releasing muscles from their strong contractions.

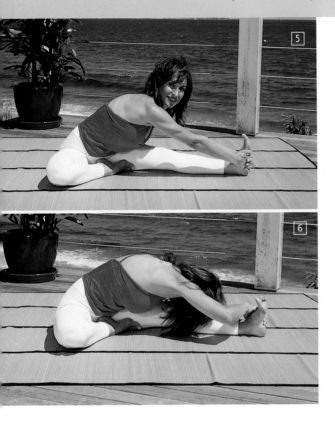

LOWER BODY ONE

Seated Head to Knee
(Seated Forward Bend—One Leg)

STRETCHES: *Hamstrings, Thighs*
IMPROVES: *Flexibility*

After a workout, this pose stretches leg muscles especially to facilitate circulation and prevent cramping.

DIRECTIONS

1 Sit with your legs outstretched and feet together, pressing down evenly on the floor with your sit bones.

2 Bend your right leg, placing the sole of your right foot against the inside of your left thigh. Keep your left knee on the floor as much as possible.

3 Inhale while raising both arms above your head as you lift and lengthen your spine forward.

4 Exhale while bending forward from your hips, followed in turn by your lower back, your middle back, and your upper back. Rest your chest as close to your knees as you can.

5 Grab the toes of your extended foot and gradually ease your body forward, clasping your hands around the sole of your foot. Hold this pose for 5 breaths.

6 Place your right hand on the outside of your left foot or ankle—wherever is the farthest you can reach. Place your left hand on the floor behind you and twist your body over, lifting and stretching out to the side. (Your ultimate goal here is for your right ear to meet your left knee. Not everyone will be able to do it the first time, but you will get better at it!) Hold this pose for 5 breaths.

7 Repeat, but do everything with the opposite leg.

Spinal Twist

STRETCHES: *Spine*

IMPROVES: *Spinal flexibility*

This pose is intended to stretch and extend your spine from top to bottom, nourishing your vertebrae (discs). Twisting poses should never be forced, and good posture should be maintained throughout. Never lead with your head, which can lead to neck strain, as we all have a tendency to pull our heads around farther and faster than may be good for them. Let your head follow the spine like the handle of a cane.

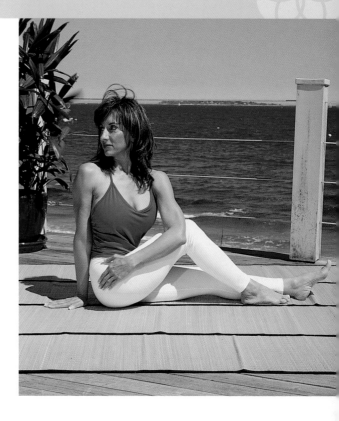

DIRECTIONS

1 Sit tall, with your spine as straight as you can get it and with both legs extended forward.

2 Raise your right knee and place your right foot on the floor; allow your left leg to remain flat on the floor.

3 Place your right hand flat on the floor behind you, not too far from your body, since this will make you lean rather than twist, compressing your spine instead of giving it a lateral stretch.

4 Raise your left arm and bring it over the right side of your right knee, bend your elbow, using resistance against your knee, and touch your thigh.

5 Inhale while extending and lengthening your spine.

6 Exhale while rotating your body farther toward the right, looking over your right shoulder. Hold this pose for 5 breaths, twisting a little farther with each exhalation.

7 Repeat on the other side, bending your left leg and twisting to your left.

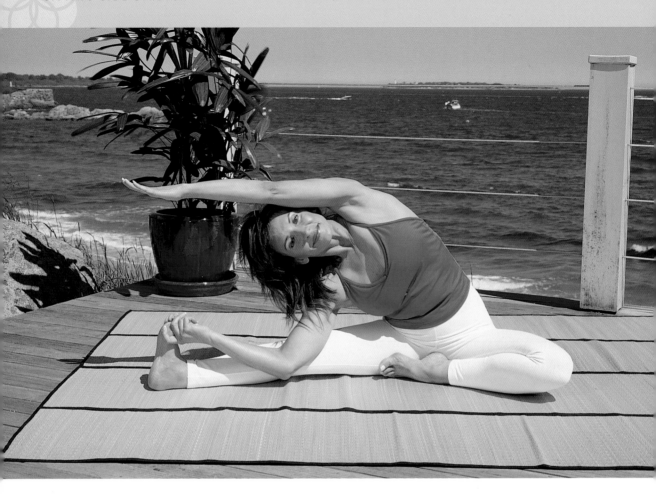

Sitting Side Stretch

STRETCHES: *Waist, Spine*

IMPROVES: *Flexibility*

This pose stretches the lateral side of the waist and at the same time stretches the spine.

DIRECTIONS

1. With your legs spread wide and your hamstring and calf muscles pressed to the floor, bend your left knee, then bend your torso over to the right and extend your left arm sideways.

2. Lean over to get a wonderful stretch to the side of the waist. Hold for 5 breaths.

3. Repeat on the other side.

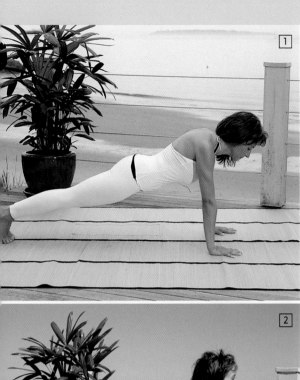

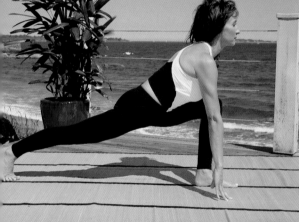

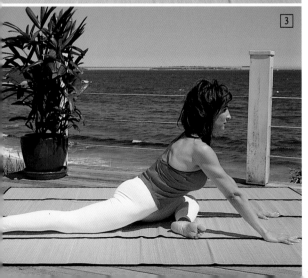

Half Pigeon
(Runner's Lunge)

STRETCHES: *Hip rotator muscles*
IMPROVES: *Flexibility*

This pose is a full hip abductor stretch, lengthening the lower muscles, releasing the periformis muscle, which is notorious for getting tight in athletes and runners.

DIRECTIONS

1   Get into the Plank Pose by placing your hands on the floor directly below your shoulders. Your fingers should be pointing forward. Extend your legs with your toes tucked under, and hold your body so it is flat.

2   Bring your left leg forward under your body, at a 90-degree angle or less, depending on the flexibility of your hips and any knee problems you might have.

3   Slowly drop your bent knee to the floor and lower your body down over the bent leg. Your body should be straight and squared forward, not twisted, and your back leg should extend straight behind you.

4   Inhale while extending your chest up to the sky.

5   Exhale while sinking your chest to the floor.

6   Bring your arms forward and hold the pose for 5 breaths.

7   Switch legs and repeat the pose.

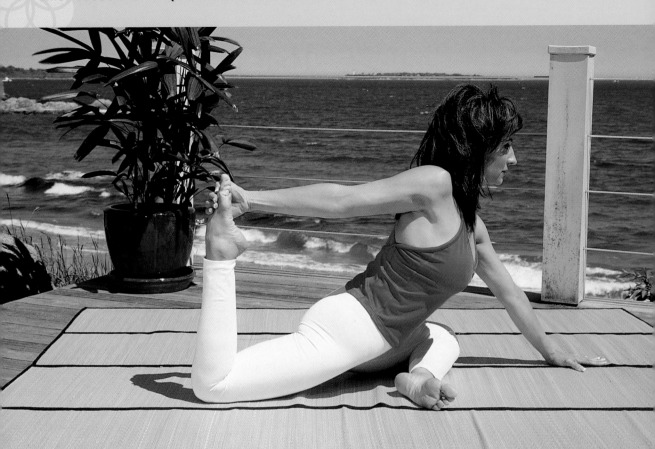

Half Pigeon with Quadricep Stretch

STRETCHES: *Quadricep muscles, Hips*
IMPROVES: *Flexibility*

DIRECTIONS

1. From the Pigeon Pose, while sitting up, bring your right arm behind you and grab hold of your right foot. Draw it in as close as you can toward your body. This will stretch your quadriceps muscle.

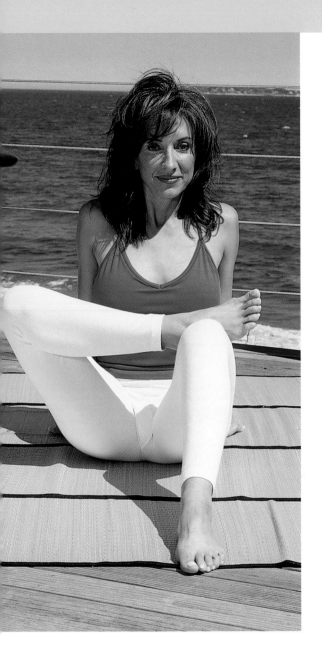

Modified Pigeon

STRETCHES: *Hip muscles*
IMPROVES: *Flexibility*

This is a modified version of the Half Pigeon Pose, especially useful for people with knee pain and those who have had knee surgery.

DIRECTIONS

1. From a seated position, set your feet flat on the floor with your knees bent.

2. Bring one foot up to the opposite thigh.

3. Set your hands on the floor behind your hips, then "walk" them in, moving your torso toward your legs until you feel a deep stretch in your buttocks.

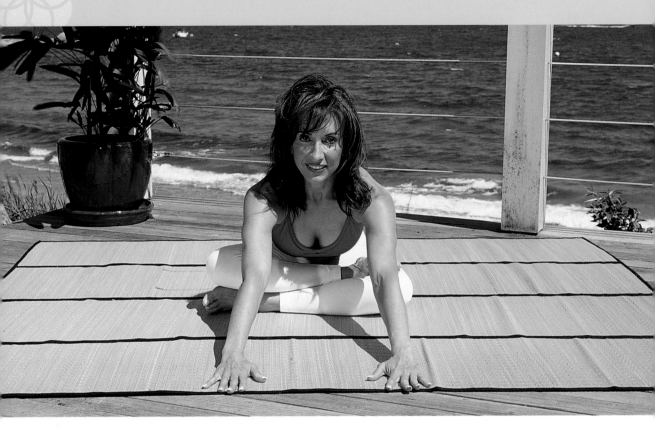

Double Pigeon

STRETCHES: *Hips*

This is a deep hip stretch that opens you up.

DIRECTIONS

1. From a seated position. Stack your right ankle on your left knee. (You can modify the pose by placing one leg in front of the other.)

2. Walk your hands forward as far as they will go. Hold this pose for 5 breaths.

3. Repeat on the other side.

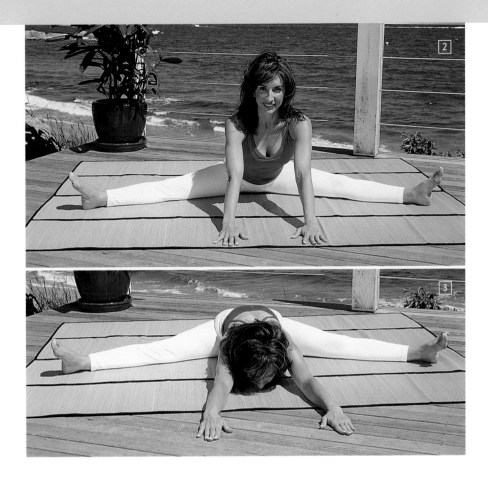

Open Angle Pose

STRETCHES: *Hamstrings*

IMPROVES: *Spinal flexibility*

This intense stretching pose provides great exercise for the hamstrings. It opens up the muscles in the inner leg and groin.

DIRECTIONS

1. Spread your legs wide apart and press your hamstring and calf muscles to the floor. Flex your feet and sit tall.

2. Stretch your arms over your head, lengthening your spine. Bend from the waist. When your hands touch the floor, gently walk them forward until you feel a good stretch. Ultimately, you will want to reach the final position, where your chest and chin rest on the floor and your arms are extended all the way to each side. If you cannot get that far initially, keep at it— every inch counts in getting more flexible!

3. Make sure your spine stays long and extended. You should be conscious of releasing your neck muscles. Hold this pose for 5 breaths.

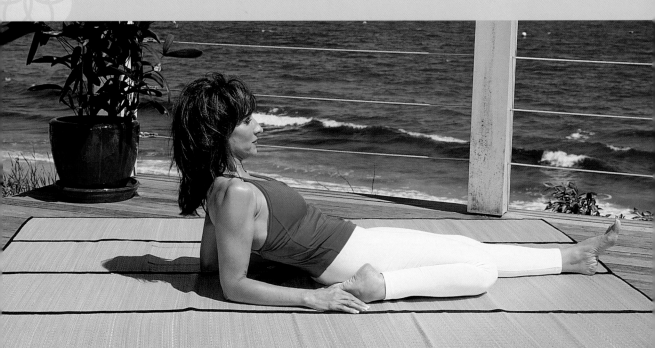

LOWER BODY TWO

Reclining Hero

STRETCHES: *Quadriceps*

IMPROVES: *Stronger and more flexible knees*

This pose produces an intense stretch in the thighs and is especially useful for people who have tight thighs from running or playing sports. The knees will also benefit by becoming stronger.

DIRECTIONS

1. Sit with one knee bent back and one leg straight in front of you.

2. Lean back on your elbows for a good stretch to your thigh. Hold this pose for 5 breaths.

3. Repeat on the other side.

CHALLENGE

To add a challenge, lie flat on the floor and bring your arms over your head onto the floor for an intense stretch.

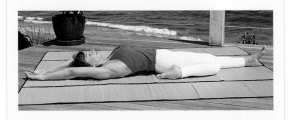

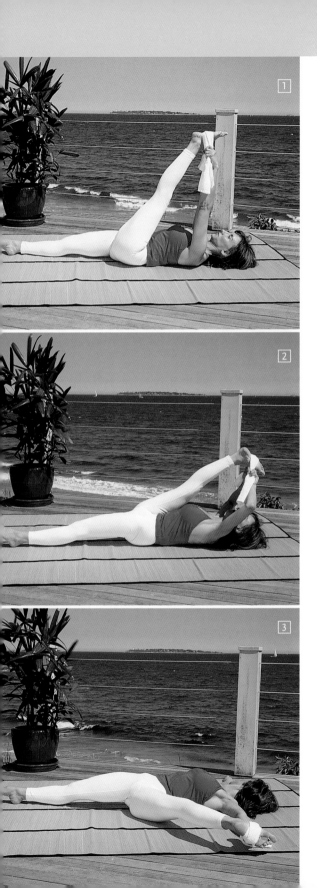

Hamstring Stretch and to the Side

This is a full-leg stretch, especially useful for improving the hamstrings and taking the leg over to the side you will be opening.

DIRECTIONS

1 Lying flat on the floor, place a small towel around your left foot.

2 Draw your straight leg in toward your body. Hold for 5 breaths.

3 Extend your leg all the way out to the side, still holding the towel around your foot with one hand. (If a towel is not long enough to get a full stretch, use a strap or a belt.) Look over your right shoulder.

4 Repeat on the other side.

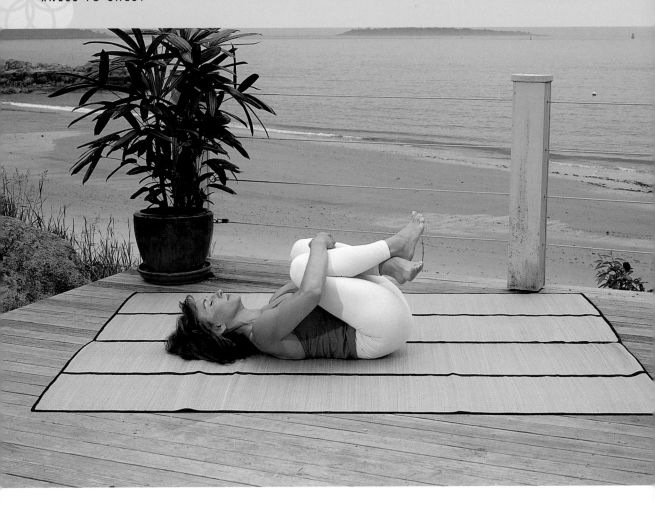

Knees to Chest

DIRECTIONS

1 Bring both knees in tight against your chest.

2 Wrap both arms around your knees in a hug, and hold for a few breaths or until you feel your spine and abdominal muscles relax.

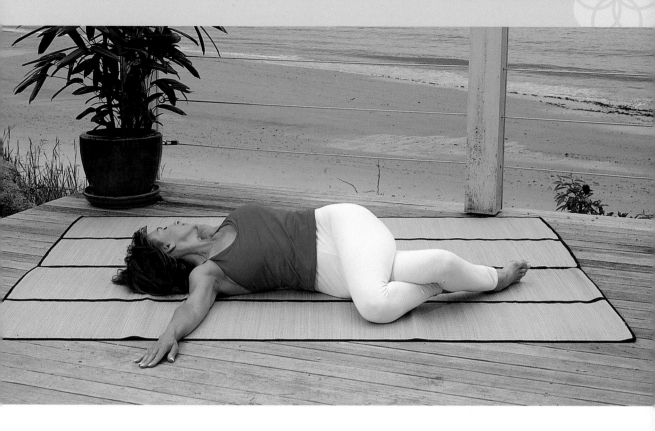

Lying Down Hip Stretch

STRENGTHENS AND TONES: *Back*
STRETCHES: *Back muscles, Hips*

This pose is actually quite relaxing and easy, gently stretching the muscles in your lower back and hips and releasing tension at the end of a complete workout.

DIRECTIONS

1. Lie flat on the floor, arms stretched out to the side and palms pressing into the floor.

2. Inhale, bending your right leg and wrapping your left thigh over your right thigh, entwining your legs and keeping your back on the floor.

3. Exhale, bringing your legs over to the right. Twist your spine to the left while turning your head to the left.

4. Slowing bring your legs back to the center. Uncross and recross your legs in the opposite direction.

5. Repeat on the opposite side.

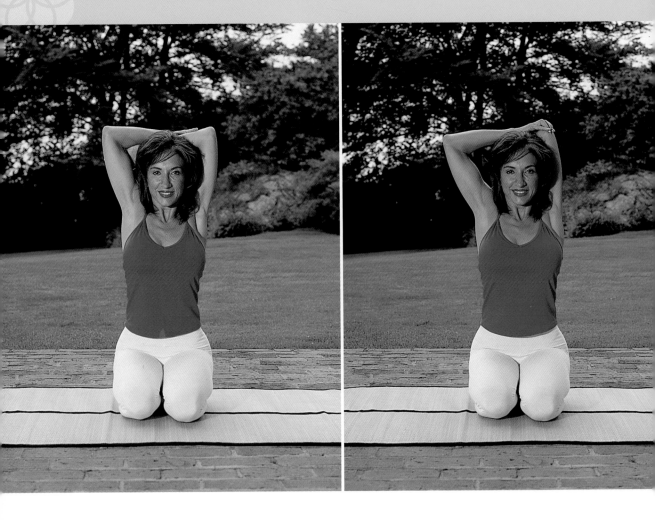

UPPER BODY ONE

Shoulder/Triceps Stretch 1

This pose stretches the triceps and the top of the shoulders.

DIRECTIONS

1. With your arms held overhead, hold the elbow of one arm with the hand of the other arm.

2. Gently pull your elbow behind your head, creating a stretch. Hold this pose for 5 breaths.

3. Repeat on the other side.

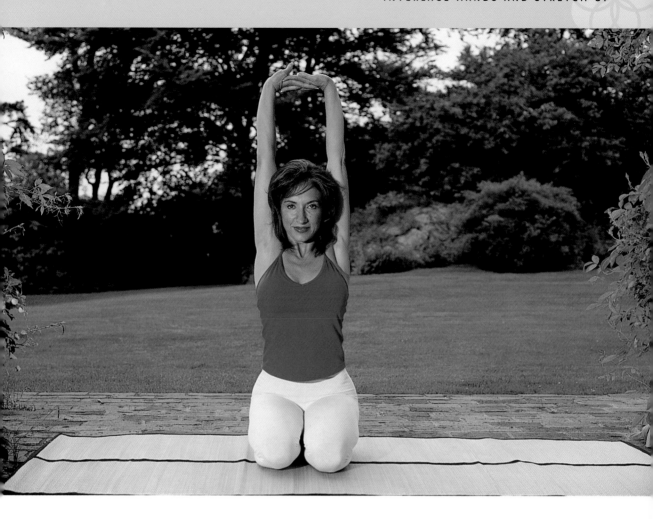

Interlace Hands and Stretch Up

This pose stretches the arms, shoulders, and upper back.

DIRECTIONS

1. Interlace your fingers above your head, with your palms facing up. Hold this pose for 5 breaths.

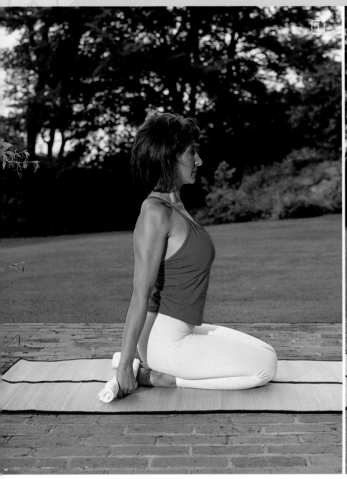
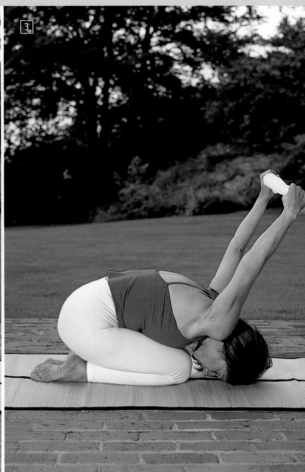

Shoulder/Triceps Stretch 2

STRETCHES: *Arms and shoulders*

DIRECTIONS

1   Hold a towel behind your back at shoulder-width distance.

2   Slowly lower your torso forward toward the floor.

3   With your forehead on the floor, extend your arms as high as they will go. Hold this pose for 5 breaths.

4   Return to a seated position.

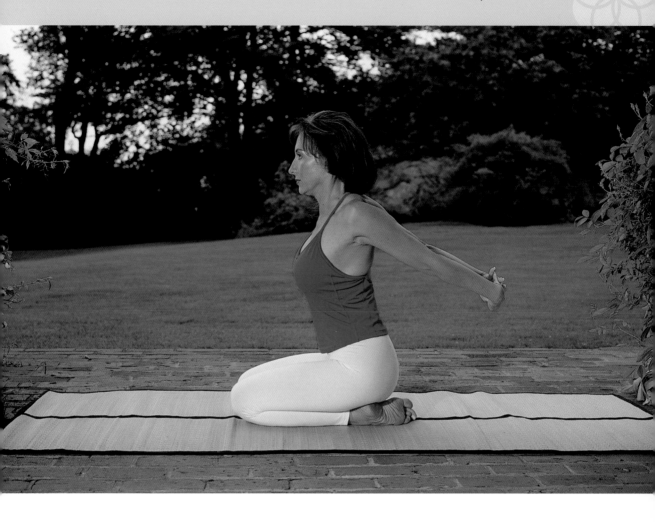

Arm/Shoulder Stretch

DIRECTIONS

1 Kneel on the floor with your spine straight. Interlace your fingers behind your back.

2 With your shoulders back and your arms straight, lift your arms as high as you can. Feel a good stretch in your arms and shoulders. Hold this pose for 5 breaths.

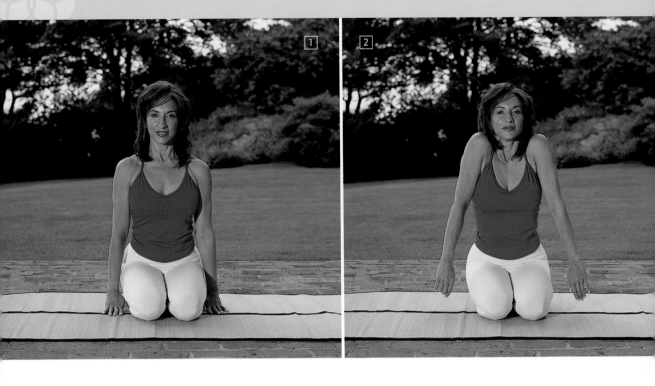

UPPER BODY TWO

Shoulder Shrugs

DIRECTIONS

1   Sit on your knees, buttocks to heels.

2   Squeeze and raise your shoulders toward your ears.

3   Quickly release.

4   Repeat this exercise 5 times.

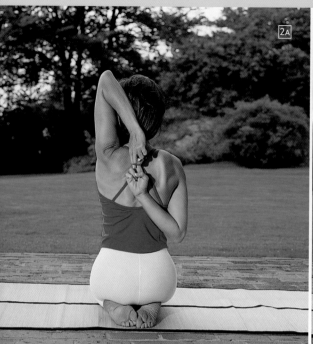
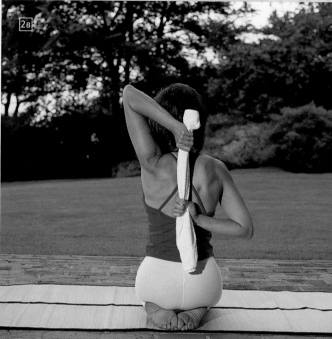

Shoulder/Arm Stretch

STRETCHES: *Neck and shoulder muscles*

Stretching following yoga poses releases tension. No place is worse to have tight muscles than in the neck and shoulders—this pose is just the trick for releasing them. This pose stretches tight neck and shoulder muscles, loosening them up for better flexibility.

DIRECTIONS

1. Sit on your knees, buttocks to heels. (Note: If this is hard on your knees, use padding or a towel, or fold over your mat. If this is still uncomfortable, perform the pose from a kneeling position.)

2. With your spine straight and erect, raise your left arm and bring it down behind your head. Bend your right arm up behind your back. Clasp your hands. (If your hands do not meet behind your back, you can use a small towel to bridge the gap, and walk your hands toward one another.)

3. Make sure your shoulders are level and your collarbones are broad. Hold this pose for 10 seconds.

4. Switch arms and repeat the pose.

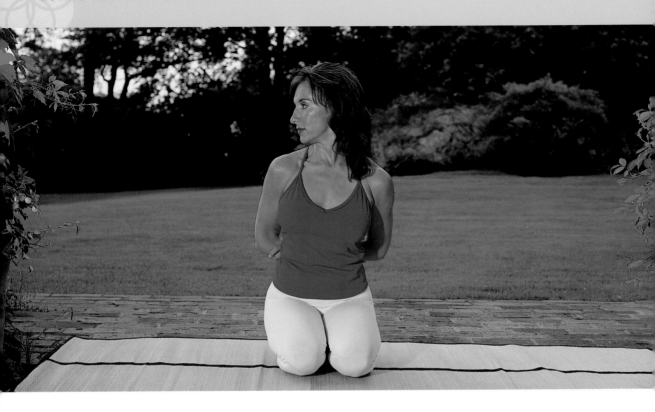

Rotate Head Side to Side

DIRECTIONS

1. Hold your elbows with opposite hands behind your back.

2. With good posture, slowly turn your head to the right, keeping your head level, and look over your right shoulder as far as you comfortably can.

3. Turn your head back to the center and repeat on the other side, being sure not to overextend.

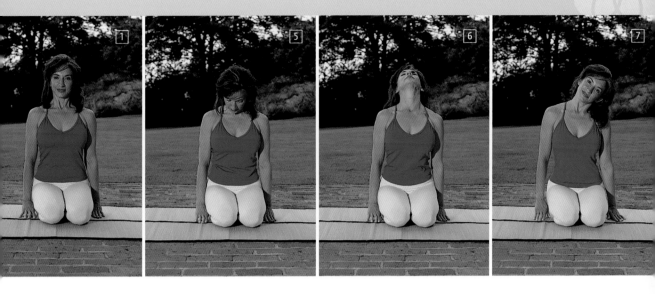

Neck and Shoulder Stretch

The Neck and Shoulder Stretch releases tension in your shoulders and upper back and rotator cuff, as well as strengthening your neck and shoulders.

DIRECTIONS

1 Sit on your knees, buttocks to heels. Pull your shoulders down and rest your arms next to your body.

2 Lift your shoulders toward your ears.

3 Rotate your shoulders backward in little circles, bringing them back to their original position. Repeat this shoulder roll 5 times.

4 Rotate your shoulders forward in little circles, bringing them back to their original position. Repeat this shoulder roll 5 times.

5 Gently lower your chin toward your chest, stretching the back of your neck.

6 Gently lower your head as far back as you can without feeling pain, stretching the front of your neck. Bring your head back up to the starting position.

7 Gently lower your head to the right, holding your shoulders away from your ears. Repeat to the other side.

8 Close your eyes and sit for a few breaths before moving to the next pose.

The Daily Program

This program is designed to coordinate the breath with the postures. One inhalation and one exhalation make one breath. In this book, five breaths equal five inhalations and five exhalations—this is what I am referring to when I mention breath during the routines.

Breathe in an unbroken rhythm through your nose, keeping your mouth closed. However, if you become oxygen deprived, you may need to open your mouth occasionally. Always remember not to hold your breath, and beware of using short, rapid breaths that will deprive you of oxygen and as a result will make you feel tired and fatigued.

Sun Salutation

The Sun Salutation is a very powerful flow of exercises that stretches and strengthens your arm and leg muscles and promotes flexibility in your ankle, knee, and hip joints. It will totally rev up your metabolism and start burning those calories!

This is really a series of poses, not a single one, done slowly and rhythmically in coordination with the breath. The individual poses are the Plank Pose, the Modified Chaturanga (developing, as your strength increases, to a Challenge Chaturanga), and the Upward Facing Dog, finishing with the Downward Facing Dog.

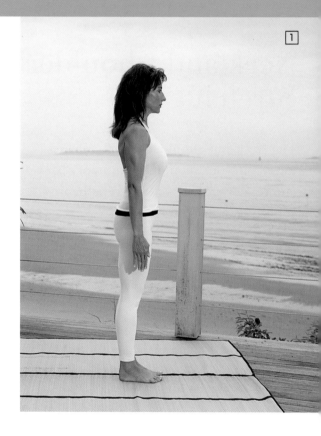

1

DIRECTIONS

1 Stand erect with your feet together and your arms by your sides.

2 Inhale, roll your arms so your palms face outward, and bring them above your head until your palms meet.

3 Exhale, and roll your arms out to the side, palms facing the floor. Gently release your head down, lengthening your spine and bending at the waist until you reach a 90-degree angle with your legs. Place your hands flat on the floor beside your feet.

4 Inhale, and lift up your head.

5 Exhale, and release your head to the floor again.

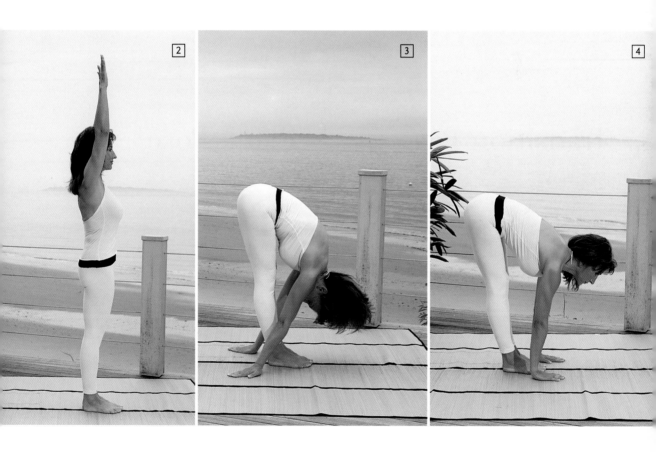

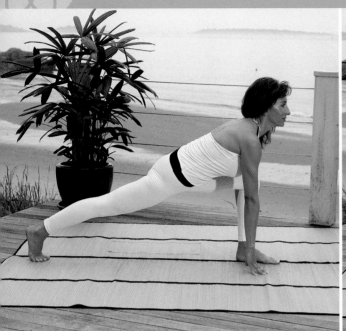 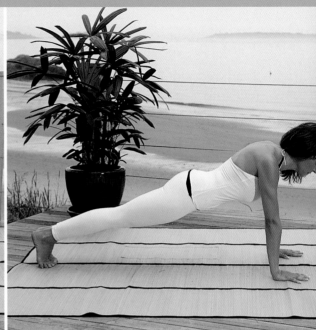

Transition Pose

DIRECTIONS

1 From the Downward Facing Dog, bring your left foot between your hands, then your right foot. Raise your torso.

Plank Pose

DIRECTIONS

1 This is a weight-bearing pose, which you can adjust into by sliding your feet behind you until you are in a position similar to a push-up, with your back straight, legs extended, toes propping you up, and hands directly beneath your shoulders, pointing forward.

2 Tuck your toes and bring yourself onto the balls of your feet, stretching your leg muscles through the heels.

3 Activate your thighs, keeping your back and body firm and flat.

4 Press firmly into your hands, and look toward the floor.

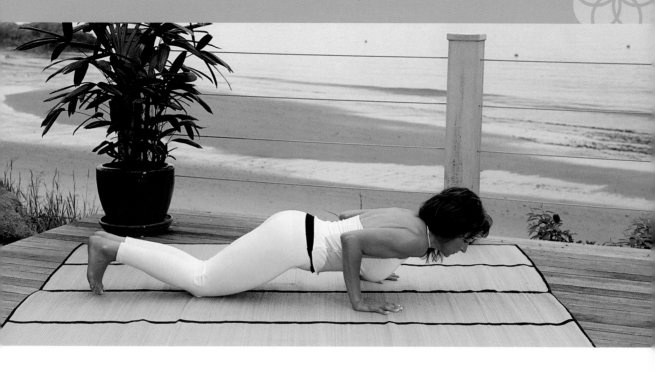

Modified Chaturanga

DIRECTIONS

1 From your position in the Plank Pose, bend your legs until your knees touch the floor, keeping your leg muscles engaged. This is the Chaturanga (a Sanskrit term for a push-up) Pose.

2 Bend your elbows directly back, keeping your arms close to your body. Look down and keep your shoulders square with the floor.

3 Continuing bending your elbows and bringing your chest toward the floor until your elbows are parallel with your shoulders. Keep your body as straight as possible. Hold this pose for 5 breaths.

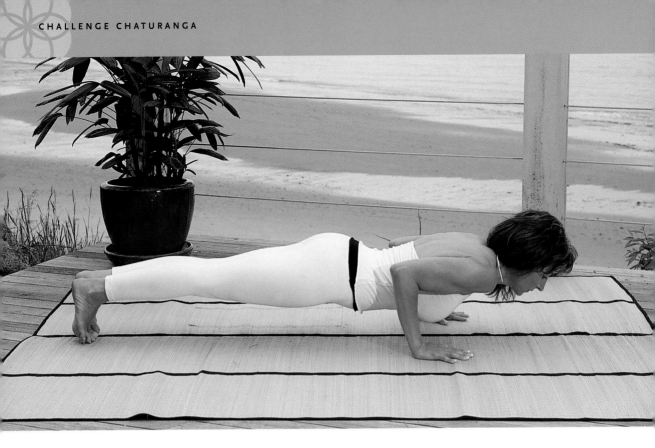

Challenge Chaturanga

As your strength increases, develop into the Challenge Chaturanga in place of the Modified Chaturanga.

DIRECTIONS

1 From your position in Plank Pose, keep your legs straight, knees off the floor, keeping your leg muscles engaged. This is the Challenge Chaturanga Pose.

2 Bend your elbows directly back, keeping your arms close to your body. Look down and keep your shoulders square with the floor.

3 Continuing bending your elbows and bringing your chest toward the floor until your elbows are parallel with your shoulders. Keep your body as straight as possible, firm and supported; don't let it sag to the floor. If this happens, place your knees to the floor in Modified Chaturanga. Hold for 5 breaths.

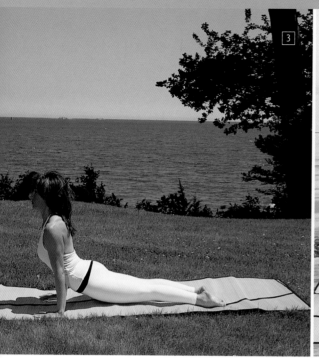
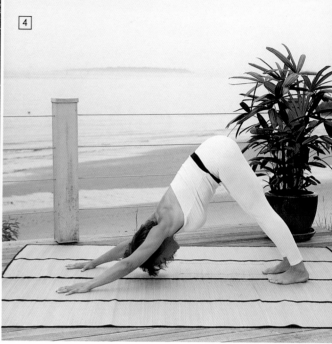

Upward Facing Dog

DIRECTIONS

1 From the Chaturanga, scoop up your chest and pull your whole body forward, rolling over the tops of your toes until the soles of your feet are facing the sky.

2 Open and lift your chest, straighten your arms, and raise your body so that only your hands and the tops of your feet support your entire body. You can try to lift your thighs by tightening them and your buttocks.

3 Arch your spine and stare directly forward, or gently drop your head back.

4 Curl up your toes, lift your hips, and stretch back into the Downward Facing Dog.

FLAB-FIGHTING FACT

The Sun Salutation stimulates all of your systems and increases circulation throughout the body while stretching and strengthening all major muscle groups. It's an excellent calorie and fat burner.

Day One

After completing our walking and warm-up routines, we are now ready to begin Day One. To help you stay motivated, start on a day that is not hectic or rushed for you—perhaps a weekend day, or a day when you do not have to be in charge of the carpool. Subsequent days should normally take thirty minutes whether you're an expert or a novice, but you should devote more time to Day One so that you can acquaint yourself with the poses and routines, and to get used to the terminology if it is new to you. Once you have become accustomed to it all, the time will fly by and you will have no problem completing an entire day's yoga workout in thirty minutes.

Each day is designed to exercise a particular body area or discipline. Day One will be Standing Strengthening Poses, and as with every day, it begins with the Sun Salutation.

Sun Salutation

This series of poses will be the first step in the process of fighting flab and starting to tone all the areas of the body.

Repeat from pages 88–93.

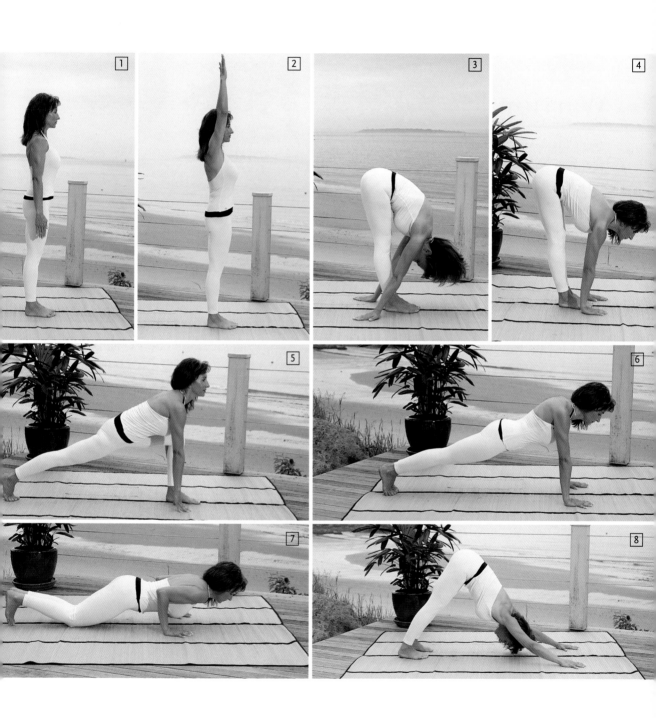

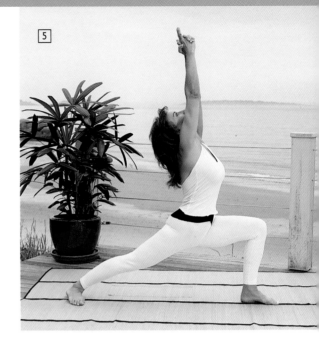

Warrior 1

STRENGTHENS AND TONES: *Thigh muscles, Glutes, Upper body*

STRETCHES: *Groin, Leg muscles*

IMPROVES: *Increased physical and mental strength, Enhanced willpower and determination*

Once you have finished with your Sun Salutation, you need to continue the exercises by adding a little bit of spice to the routine. The Warrior 1 Pose continues from the Sun Salutation. It is called a Warrior pose, like many of the subsequent poses, because of the stance's aggressive appearance—one leg in front of the other, like a stance of victory for a legendary Hindu warrior. You will do it first with the left leg in front; then repeat with the right leg in front.

DIRECTIONS

1. From the Downward Facing Dog position, bend your left knee and bring your left foot forward until it is flat on the ground between your hands. (If you have balance problems early on, you may stand and position yourself into the pose.)

2. Leave your right foot on the floor behind you, turning it outward and to a 45-degree angle, like a backstop.

3. Check the position of your feet—your body should be midway between them— about three feet apart, so that when your arms are spread open, each foot is directly below one set of fingertips.

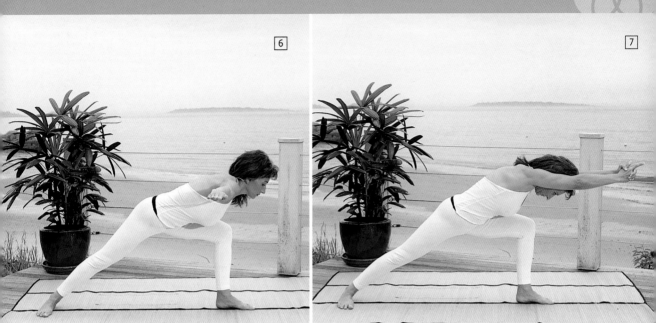

4   Square your hips forward, pointing your front foot directly ahead and making sure your heels are aligned.

5   Raise your arms over your head, interlace your hands, index fingers pointing upwards, and look towards your hands. Bend your left knee until it is directly above your ankle, forming a 90-degree angle.

6   We are injecting movement into this pose here. Bend forward from the waist, gazing toward the ground, arm out to the sides. Hold, then return to the starting position.

7   Repeat steps 5 and 6, reaching upward with your arms again, then bending forward from your waist with your arms forward.

8   Bring your hands flat on each side of your left foot, and bring your leg behind you, returning to the Plank Pose.

From the Plank Pose, the Warrior 1 continues with a Modified Sun Salutation. Position your hands directly below your shoulders, fingers facing forward.

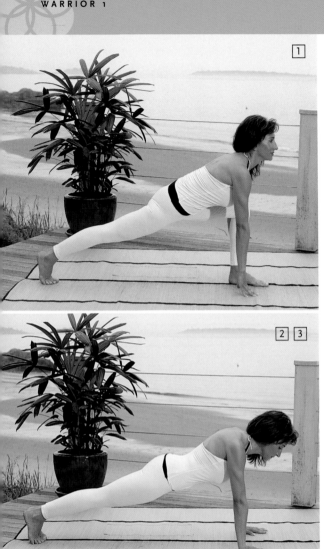

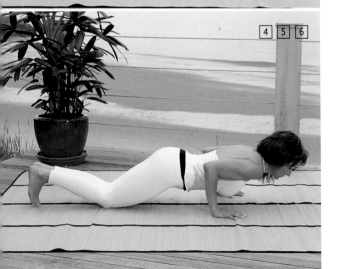

1 Begin in Transition Pose (page 55).

2 Tuck your toes and bring yourself onto the balls of your feet, stretching your leg muscles through the heels. Activate your thighs, keeping your back and body firm and flat.

3 Press firmly into your hands, and look toward the floor.

4 Bend your legs until your knees touch the floor, keeping your leg muscles engaged.

5 Bend your elbows directly back, keeping your arms close to your body. Look down and keep your shoulders square with the floor.

6 Continue bending your elbows and bringing your chest toward the floor until your elbows are parallel with your shoulders. Keep your body as straight as possible. Hold this pose for 5 breaths.

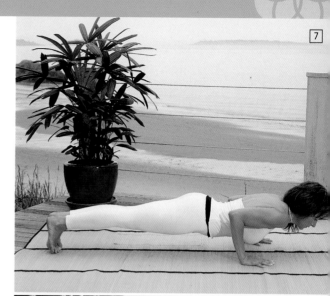

7 If you have mastered the Challenge Chaturanga, you can perform that here. Repeat 5 and 6 with your knees off the floor.

8 Scoop up your chest and pull your whole body forward, rolling over the tops of your toes until the soles of your feet are facing the sky in the Upward Facing Dog position. Open and lift your chest, straighten your arms, and raise your body so that only your hands and the tops of your feet support your entire body. You can try to lift your thighs by tightening them and your buttocks.

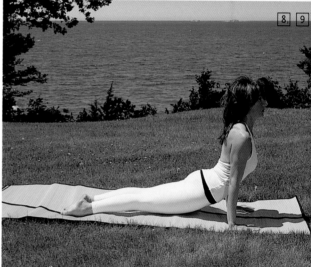

9 Arch your spine and stare directly forward, or gently drop your head back.

10 Curl up your toes, lift your hips, and stretch back into the Downward Facing Dog Pose.

FLAB-FIGHTING FACT

This pose will strengthen and tone the lower body and the upper body, reducing fat cells in problem areas like the thighs and torso.

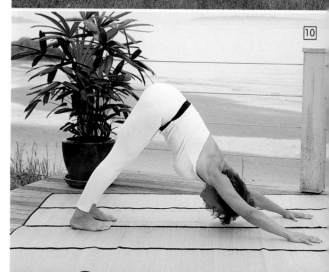

Warrior 2

STRENGTHENS AND TONES: *Thigh muscles, Glutes, Upper body*

STRETCHES: *Chest, Adductors*

IMPROVES: *Focus and discipline*

Warrior 2 rejuvenates and increases flexibility. To perform it correctly, make sure your hips are properly aligned and your lunge is deep.

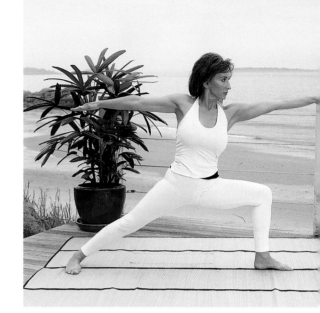

DIRECTIONS

1 Starting from the Downward Facing Dog position, bend your left knee and bring your left foot forward until it is flat on the ground between your hands. (As with Warrior 1, if you have balance problems early on, you may stand and position yourself into the pose.)

2 Leave your right foot flat on the floor. Check the position of your feet—your body should be midway between them—about three feet apart, so that when your arms are spread open each foot is directly below one set of fingertips.

3 Square your hips forward.

4 Raise your arms to shoulder height, with your palms facing the floor, and rotate your torso so that your arms are aligned with your body and legs.

5 Bend your left knee until it is directly above your ankle, forming a 90-degree angle, and lower yourself into a lunge position. (You can adjust slightly to achieve the pose correctly.) Keep your hips aligned.

6 Turn your head to the left, looking past your left hand. Hold this pose for 5 breaths.

FLAB-FIGHTING FACT

All Warrior poses fight flab by toning and shaping thighs and glutes.

Reverse Warrior

STRENGTHENS AND TONES: *Thigh muscles, Glutes*
STRETCHES: *Adductors, Stretches and lengthens the spine, Front side of the body*
IMPROVES: *Flexibility of the spine*

As you think about the name of each yoga pose when you do it, you should get a sense of what you are trying to accomplish. The Reverse Warrior is a pose of victory, of strength—of a warrior. It is a beginner's stance that looks just like you would imagine it would, giving you a sturdy yet graceful appearance. It will improve your balance and leave you refreshed and confident.

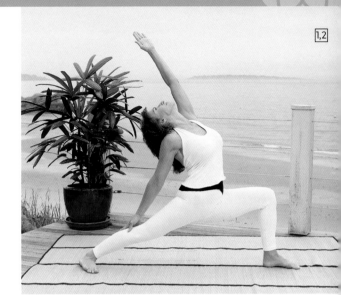

DIRECTIONS

1. From Warrior 2, inhale, raising your left arm toward the sky and sliding your right arm down your right leg while gently bending backward at the waist.

2. Exhale, slowly moving your head up and back.

3. Let your lower body sink into the pose as you lift your upper body toward the sky. Hold this pose for 5 breaths.

4. Return to the Warrior 2 Pose, holding your arms at shoulder length with your palms facing the ground. Do not move the lower body or legs. Hold for 5 breaths.

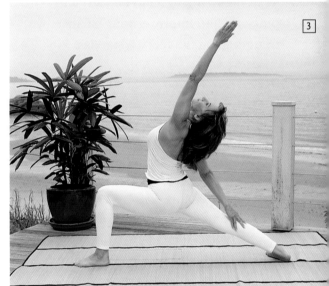

FLAB-FIGHTING FACT
The Reverse Warrior builds tremendous strength in your body while toning and reshaping your legs. It is the pose for flab-free legs and thighs!

Triangle Pose

STRENGTHENS AND TONES: *Back, Hamstrings, Thigh muscles, Calf muscles*
STRETCHES: *Hamstrings, Waist and sides of torso, Expands your chest*
IMPROVES: *Balance, Spinal flexibility*

This pose looks like what it sounds like—a big triangle. It lengthens and stretches the spine and also improves your balance by strengthening the feet and ankles.

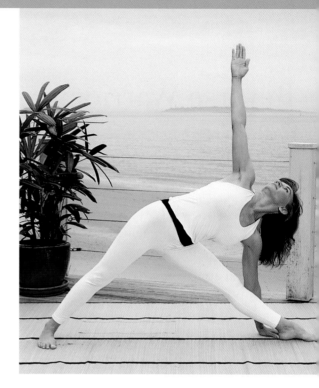

DIRECTIONS

1 From the prior Warrior 2 Pose, straighten the left front leg and extend your arms straight out from your shoulders, keeping your quadriceps actively contracted.

2 Inhale, shifting your torso to the left, placing your left hand flat on the floor on the outside of your left foot. If you can't reach the floor, grab hold of your ankle or shin.

3 Reach your right arm up toward the sky, extending your spine. Open your chest and look up toward your arm. Lengthen your head away from your tailbone, positioning your torso as parallel to the floor as possible.

4 Exhale, and open up your chest as far as you can toward the sky, shifting your body weight toward the back of your heel. Hold this pose for 5 breaths.

FLAB-FIGHTING FACT

This pose keeps your back in shape, working the muscles there. Flab can appear in odd places, and a thickness in the back is one of the hardest to defeat—but not when you master this pose!

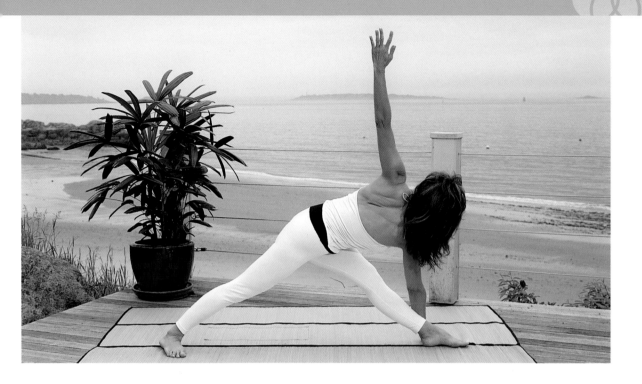

Revolved Triangle

STRENGTHENS AND TONES: *Legs, Obliques, Waist*
STRETCHES: *Spine, Hips, Hamstrings*
IMPROVES: *Balance, Overall flexibility*

This pose progresses you through the Triangle Sequence by adding flexibility.

DIRECTIONS

1 While still in the Triangle Pose, inhale and twist your torso to the left, rotating your right arm all the way over to the outside of your left foot, or modify by reaching for your leg or shin.

2 Pull your right hip back as you look up and over your left shoulder.

3 Exhale, stretching your arms and shoulders away from your breastbone and extending your left arm toward the sky. Hold this pose for 5 breaths.

4 Repeat the Triangle Pose and Revolved Triangle Pose, reversing your legs.

FLAB-FIGHTING FACT

The Triangle Pose tones hamstring, thigh, and calf muscles, and creates even more flexibility for the spine. It incorporates many toning elements and full expression of movement to fight the cottage cheese effect of flab.

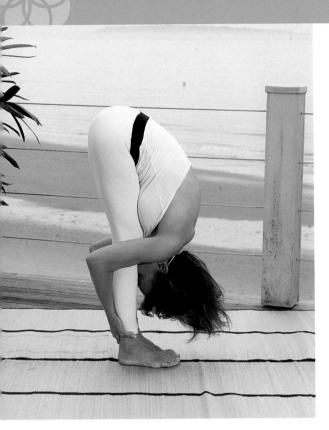

Standing Forward Bend

STRENGTHENS AND TONES: *Back*

STRETCHES: *Hamstrings, Back—opens every vertebra in the spine*

IMPROVES: *Flexibility throughout the body*

If you have ever envied ballet dancers' ability to bend gracefully, this is the pose that will let you achieve the same flexibility. It is known as an inverted posture. It stretches all major muscles and promotes overall body health.

DIRECTIONS

1 From the Revolved Triangle Pose (with your left foot forward), bend your left knee and bring each hand around to the opposite sides of your foot. Bring your right foot forward and straighten out your legs.

2 Bring your arms out to your sides, and pull your hands toward your heart center, standing upright.

3 Inhale, lifting your arms over your head.

4 Exhale, folding your body forward from the hips (not from the middle of the back), keeping your spine straight. Relax your hip joints so that your body bends without your spine curving. Place your hands on the floor next to your feet; if you cannot do that, start out by grabbing hold of your shins or ankles.

5 Lift your buttocks and lower your head to your shins. Relax your abdominal muscles, easing into the pose. (Don't force it.) Hold for 5 breaths.

FLAB-FIGHTING FACT

This pose increases blood flow to your head for clearer, more positive thinking. It also acts to fight fat in the abdomen.

Sun Salutation

Repeat from pages 88–93.

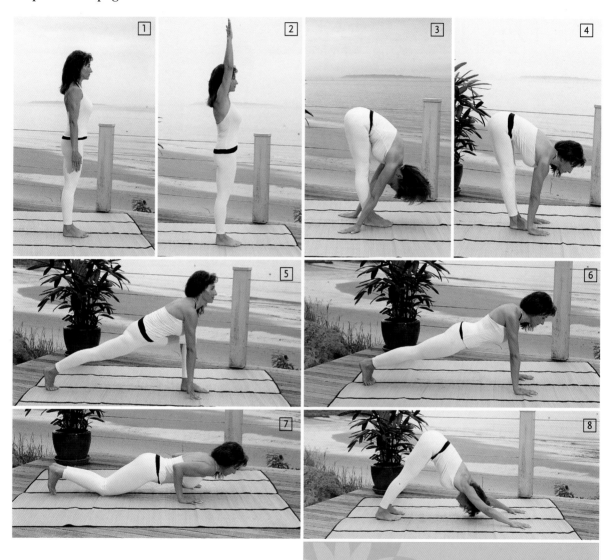

Savasana

Repeat from page 40.

FLAB-FIGHTING FACT

Its versatility and application make Sun Salutation one of the most useful methods of inducing a healthy, vigorous, and active life. The application of these positions and rhythm is transforming for the mind and the body.

Day Two

Yoga can be exhausting if you have never done anything active before, but unlike many other exercises, on the second day of this program you will probably find that you are not sore. That's because of the stretching, which prevents soreness.

Day Two begins our program of Balancing Poses. Balancing postures help to develop and maintain physical and mental equilibrium. Balance is strongly affected by your emotional state, so by learning to balance the body, you can learn how to calm the mind. These poses will also improve as you strengthen the muscles in your legs and gain flexibility in the knees and ankles. They will tighten and tone your thighs, hips, buttocks, and arms.

For those familiar with yoga, most of the poses on this day will not seem familiar to you. That is because these are not "traditional" poses, but ones I have designed specifically to combat flab.

Sun Salutation

Repeat from pages 88–93.

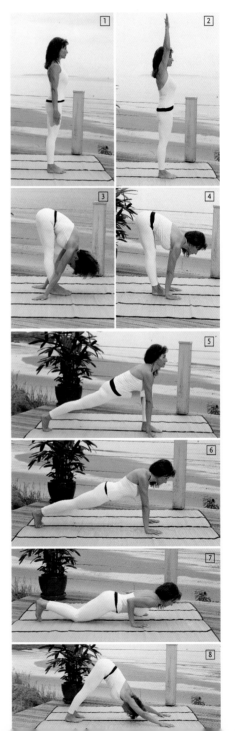

Standing, Balancing, and Toning Pose

STRENGTHENS AND TONES: *All leg muscles, Ankles, Knee joints*
STRETCHES: *Hip joints*
IMPROVES: *Balance*

This pose is equivalent to a martial arts pose because it balances and strengthens the mind and body. At the same time, it will sculpt and tone every muscle from the waist down.

DIRECTIONS

1. From a standing position, straighten your spine, contracting your abdominal muscles as if doing a sit-up.

2. Stretch your arms out in front of you, shoulder-width apart and palms facing the ground at shoulder level. Hold them there, using the muscles in your arms to point your fingers.

3. Bend your left leg at the knee and lift your right leg out to the side—straighten and lift as high as you can. Hold the pose for 10 breaths.

4. Bring the leg down and repeat on the other side for 10 breaths.

FLAB-FIGHTING FACT

This pose will strengthen the arm, hip, and leg muscles and ankles, and slim down those areas.

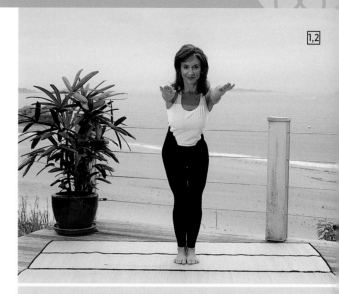

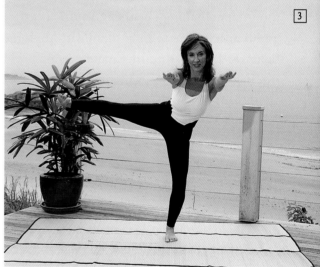

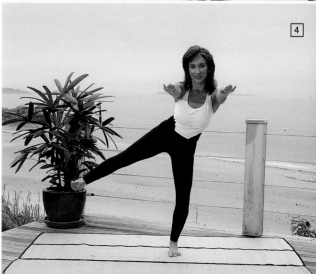

Leg Crossover Balancing Pose

STRENGTHENS AND TONES: *All leg muscles, Glutes and thighs*
STRETCHES: *Hip muscles*
IMPROVES: *Hip flexibility*

I created this pose specifically for my mountain-climbing clients in America and South Africa, to help them with their balance. The pose approximates sitting the half-lotus position while standing up.

DIRECTIONS

1. From the standing position, bring your hands together in prayer position. Gaze at a point in front of you.

2. Bend your right leg at the knee and raise your right ankle to your left thigh. Lower your body down as far as you can. Hold this pose for 10 breaths.

3. Come back to standing position still with your ankle touching your thigh. Lower once again and hold for another 10 breaths.

4. Repeat on the other side.

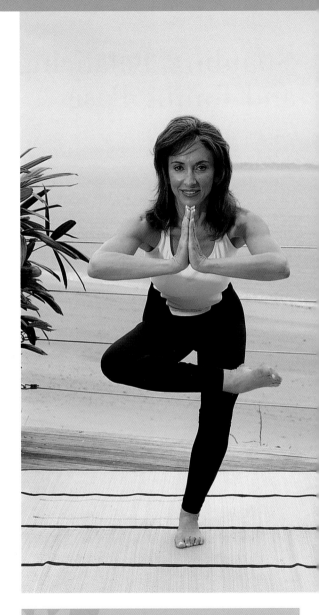

FLAB-FIGHTING FACT
You will feel the fat in your glutes and thighs fall off as you firm and tone. It slims down your backside!

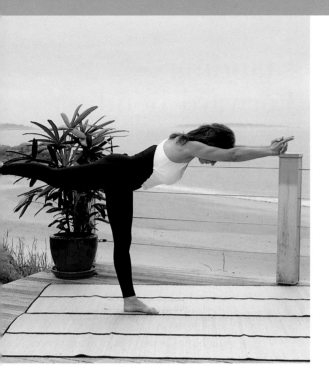

Warrior 3

STRENGTHENS AND TONES: *Arms, Hips, Legs*
STRETCHES: *Relaxes lower back*
IMPROVES: *Balance*

This is a traditional yoga pose that is physically and mentally demanding to maintain balance. It is a strong pose that will strengthen and tone all the muscles of the arms, hips, buttocks, and legs.

DIRECTIONS

1 From Leg Crossover Balancing Pose, come to a standing position, raise your arms directly in line with your head, interlocking your fingers and pointing them forward.

2 Bend forward slowly from the hips, keeping your torso, head, and arms in a straight line.

3 At the same time, raise your right leg straight back, keeping it in line with your torso. The body should pivot from the left hip joint. In the final position, the right leg, torso, head, and arms are all in one straight, horizontal line. The standing left leg is straight and vertical.

4 Focus your gaze on your hands or on the floor. Hold this pose for 10 breaths and then slowly return to the starting position.

CAUTION: *If this pulls on the lower back, bend the standing leg.*

5 Repeat Leg Crossover Balancing Pose and Warrior 3 on the opposite side.

FLAB-FIGHTING FACT

This pose develops control of the body and mental concentration. It will balance the nervous system and create more mental discipline, which will help you stick to a sensible diet and maintain your yoga program.

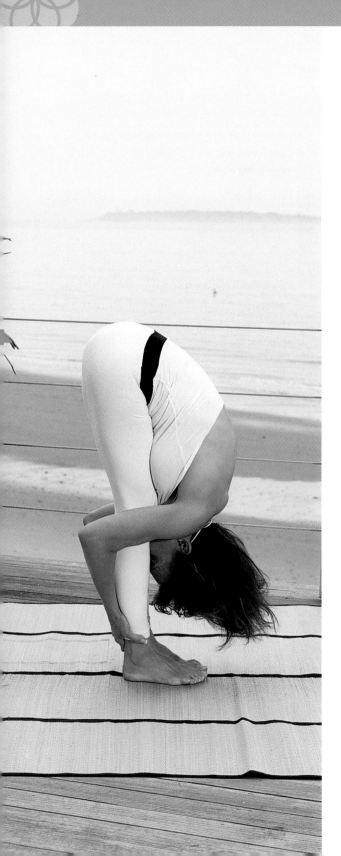

Standing Forward Bend

STRENGTHENS AND TONES: *Back*
STRETCHES: *Hamstrings, Back—opens every vertebra in the spine*
IMPROVES: *Flexibility throughout the body*

DIRECTIONS

1. From the Warrior 3 Pose, come to a standing position.

2. Bring your arms out to your sides, and pull your hands toward your heart center, standing upright.

3. Inhale, lifting your arms over your head.

4. Exhale, folding your body forward from the hips (not from the middle of the back), keeping your spine straight. Relax your hip joints so that your body bends without your spine curving. Place your hands on the floor next to your feet; if you cannot do that, start out by grabbing hold of your shins or ankles.

5. Lift your buttocks and lower your head to your shins. Relax your abdominal muscles, easing into the pose. (Don't force it.) Hold for 5 breaths.

FLAB-FIGHTING FACT

This pose increases blood flow to your head for clearer, more positive thinking. It also fights fat in the abdomen.

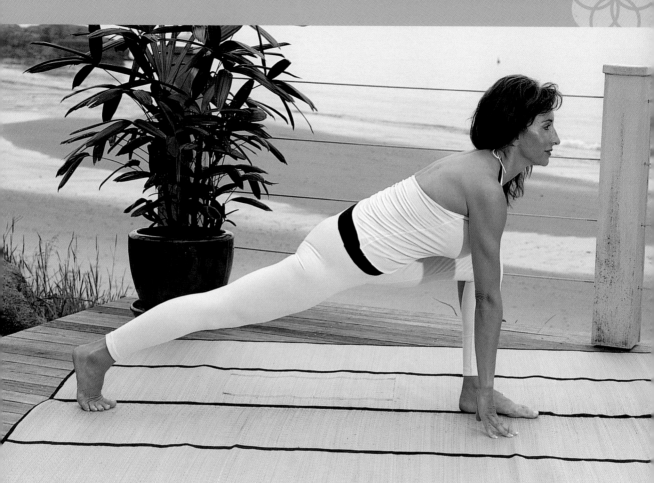

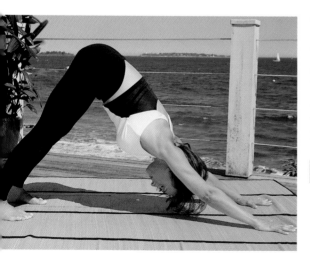

Transition into Downward Facing Dog

DIRECTIONS

1. From Standing Forward Bend, bring your left leg back and right leg back into Downward Facing Dog. Hold for 5 breaths.

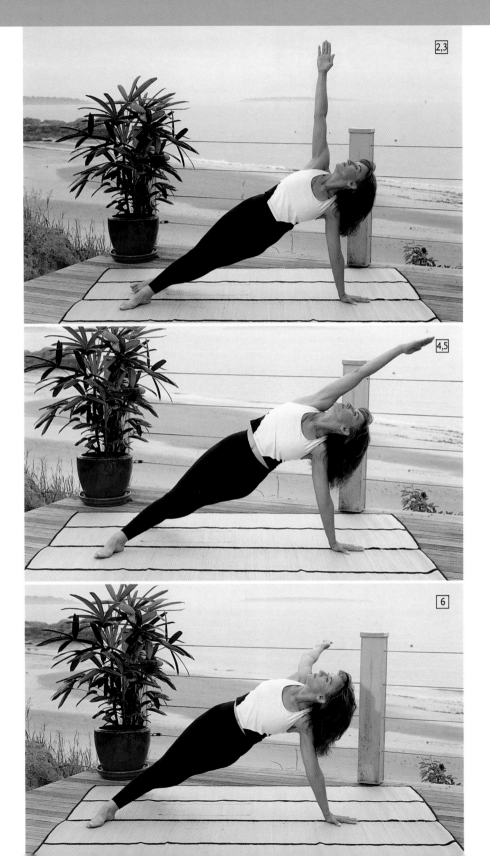

Side Plank Pose

STRENGTHENS AND TONES: *Arms and shoulders, Legs*
STRETCHES: *Obliques*
IMPROVES: *Coordination*

This pose challenges the body more than the regular Plank Pose does because your knees are never in contact with the floor. This creates more intense toning and strengthening.

FLAB-FIGHTING FACT

This activity reshapes the arms and shoulders, tightening and defining muscles for a sculpted, muscular look.

DIRECTIONS

1. From the Downward Facing Dog, transition into the Plank Pose.

2. Roll your toes to your left side, balancing on the sides your feet, one foot in front of the other, so that your inner thighs are touching one another.

3. Make sure your left hand is supporting you, directly underneath your shoulder. Raise your right hand toward the sky.
Gaze up at your right arm or directly in front of you.

4. Align your upper hip directly over your lower hip. Your heels, hips, and shoulders should also be in line.

5. Extend your right arm and reach over your head.

6. Now open your chest by bringing your right arm all the way out to the side. Hold this pose for 5 breaths. If your supporting arm wobbles intensely, you can modify the pose by lowering your left knee to the floor until you build up more strength.

7. Release your knees to the floor and get onto all fours.

8. Stretch into the Child's Pose.

9. Repeat on the other side.

Child's Pose— Arms Forward

Begin in Child's Pose but stretch your arms out in front of you. Relax your neck muscles, walking your fingers out to get a stretch, and relax into pose. (See page 146.)

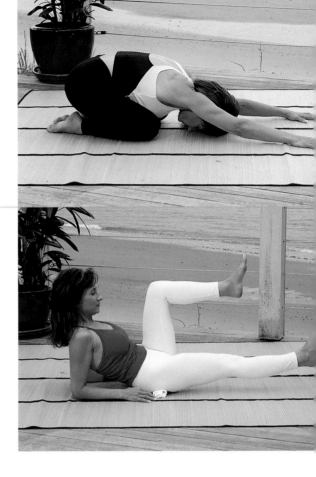

Abdominal Bicycle

STRENGTHENS AND TONES: *Abdominals (rectus abdominis)*

IMPROVES: *Stabilization of the spine, protecting it from injury*

In traditional yoga, abdominal exercises are not a main focus. But when you want to fight flab, building those abs can really get you on your way.

DIRECTIONS

1 Begin this pose while lying on your back; use your elbows to support your lower back.

2 Inhale while lifting your feet about six inches off the ground.

3 Exhale, extending your right leg by straightening your right knee and retracting your left leg by bending your left knee.

4 Alternating legs, extend and retract as if you were riding a bicycle.

5 You can add an optional element by rolling a small, thin towel and placing it where your buttocks meet the floor. This helps to isolate the abdominal muscles.

6 Practice 3 sets of 10.

FLAB-FIGHTING FACT

This "abdominal bicycle" strengthens and defines the muscles of the abdomen, decreasing fat cells in that area.

Sun Salutation

Repeat from pages 88–93.

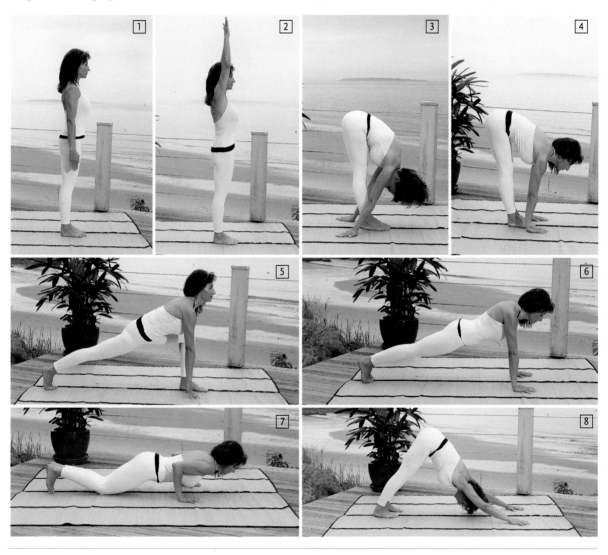

Savasana

Repeat from page 40.

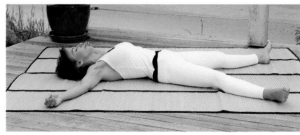

3

Day Three

*All the poses in Day Three are Twisting
Poses—full-body poses that open, stretch,
and strengthen the whole body and integrate
it as one unit. These are especially useful for
strengthening the lower body as well as
increasing your cardiovascular health. You
will cultivate balance and coordination,
and strengthen the muscles that stabilize the
knees and sculpt your legs.*

Sun Salutation

Repeat from pages 88–93.

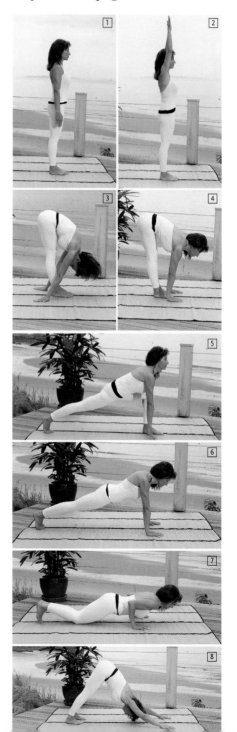

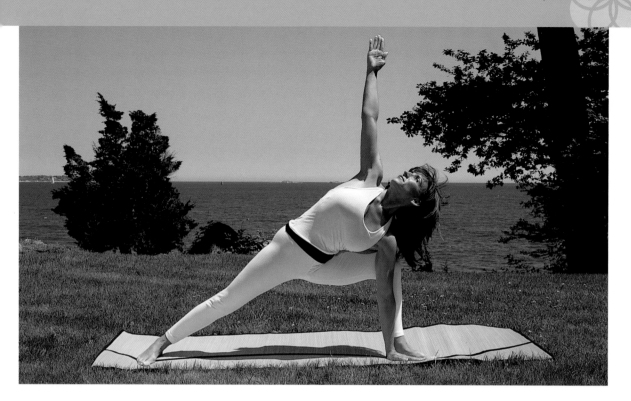

Extended Side Angle Pose

STRENGTHENS AND TONES: *Legs and thighs, Ankles and knees*

STRETCHES: *Opens the chest, Pectoral minor muscles*

IMPROVES: *Balance and coordination*

This diagonal stretch works the upper body in a dynamic fashion while strengthening and reshaping the thighs.

DIRECTIONS

1. From the Warrior 2 position, inhale while leaning toward your left, placing your left elbow in front of your left knee.

2. Lift your right arm in line with your head, forming a straight line from your heel all the way up toward the sky.

3. Exhale, and turn your head upward, looking under your right arm and toward the sky, or toward the floor if you have a neck injury. Hold this pose for 5 breaths. Repeat on the other side.

FLAB-FIGHTING FACT

This pose promotes the tightening, toning, and reshaping of your legs, thighs, and the midsection of your body.

Extended Side Angle Wraparound ("Arms Bound")

STRENGTHENS AND TONES: *Legs and thighs, Ankles and knees*
STRETCHES: *Opens the chest, Pectoral minor muscles*
IMPROVES: *Balance and coordination*

"Arms bound" means this is a challenge pose that requires you to reach behind you and hook your hands. From the modified Extended Side Angle Pose, reach behind you with both hands.

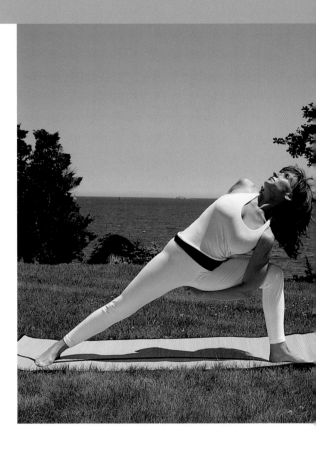

DIRECTIONS

1 From the Extended Side Angle Pose, bend your right elbow back behind you and reach through your legs with your left hand. Try to hook your hands or wrist without compromising the pose.

CAUTION: *Be careful not to let your torso drop forward—just wrap your arms around the back of you and maintain the same position.*

2 You can modify the pose by placing a towel between your hands.

3 Hold for 10 breaths.

4 Stay in this pose as we transition into the Revolving Side Angle Lunge.

FLAB-FIGHTING FACT
This pose promotes the tightening, toning, and reshaping of the legs, thighs, and midsection of the body.

Revolving Side Angle Lunge

STRENGTHENS AND TONES: *Lower body*
STRETCHES: *Pectoral minor muscles in the chest,*
Opens up the chest
IMPROVES: *Health of the internal organs*

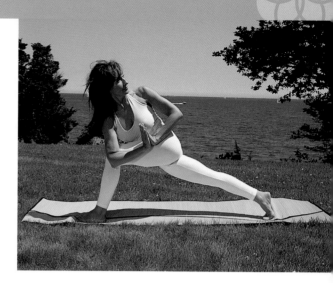

This twisting pose significantly contributes to overall internal well-being. (Twisting the torso improves the efficiency and health of the glands, circulatory system, and the muscles.) It stretches and flexes your spine without the dangers of high-impact workouts, and is wonderful for building and toning the legs and thighs.

DIRECTIONS

1. From Extended Side Angle Wraparound, lift your right heel off the floor as you square your hips forward, still bending the left knee, keeping the right leg straight as can be. If balance is a problem here, you can leave your right foot flat and keep it turned out to a 45-degree angle.

2. Rotate your right elbow around to the outside of your left thigh. Bring your hands together in a Prayer Position.

3. Keep your back leg straight and contracted. Hold for 5 breaths.

4. Straighten your arms by raising them upward, bringing your left hand to the floor (on the outside of your left foot) and lifting your right hand to the sky. You can look up, center, or to the floor. (If you cannot bring your hand to the outside of your foot, place it on the floor to the inside of your front foot, directly under your shoulder.) Hold for 5 breaths.

FLAB-FIGHTING FACT

This is a great exercise for reducing waistline fat by working the muscles on the sides of your waist.

CHALLENGE
Revolving Side Angle Lunge Wrap Around

Bend your right elbow back behind you and reach through your legs with your left hand; try and hook your hands or wrists. Hold for 5 breaths.

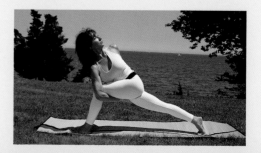

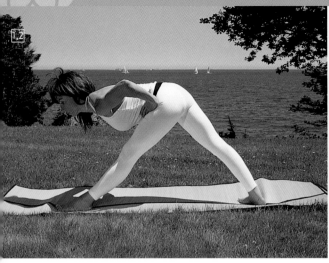

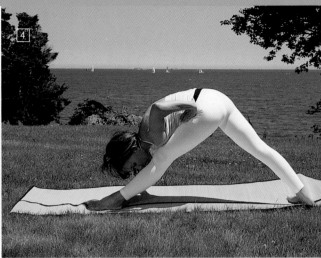

Standing Head to Knee (One Leg) Pose

STRENGTHENS AND TONES: *Sciatic nerves,*
   Tendons of the legs
STRETCHES: *Legs, particularly the hamstrings, Hips*
IMPROVES: *Flexibility*

This is a Standing Pose that stretches the hamstrings.

DIRECTIONS

1. Place your hands on your waist. From the Revolved Side Angle Pose, bring your torso up and straighten out both legs, keeping your thighs active. The toes of your front foot should face forward, and your back foot should remain still, at a 45-degree angle.

2. Square your hips and shoulders forward.

3. Inhale, and lengthen through your entire spine, from your tailbone to your head.

4. Exhale, bending your body forward from the hips. Lift your tailbone up toward the sky, leading with your chest toward your leg and surrendering your head. Keep your head and spine in a straight line. Release your neck muscles, keeping them soft. Hold this pose for 5 breaths.

5. Repeat the following poses on the opposite side:
   1. Extended Side Angle Pose
   2. Extended Side Angle Wraparound
   3. Revolving Side Angle Lunge

Sun Salutation

Repeat from pages 88–93.

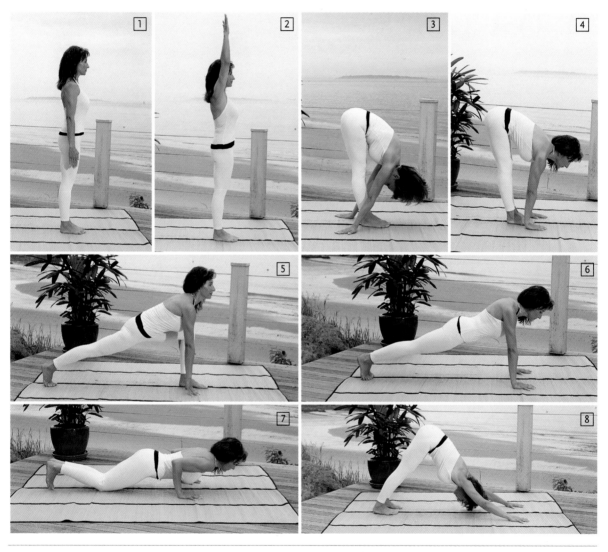

Savasana

Repeat from page 40.

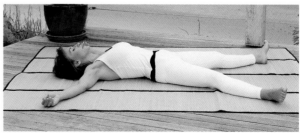

Day Four

The Back Strengthening Poses of Day Four attack a particularly problematic area of the body flab-wise—the thickness in your lower back. Personally, I never had any back muscles before I started doing yoga eight years ago. Now my back is sculpted like a dancer's. Yours can be, too! All the Back Strengthening Poses do just that—they strengthen and condition every muscle on the back side of the body. These poses relax and eliminate tension, aches, and pains in the back. Working and conditioning the muscles of the back will tone and sculpt them and at the same time remove the excess fat in that area.

Sun Salutation

Repeat from pages 88–93.

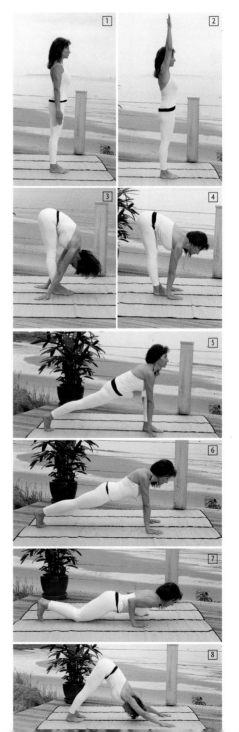

Spinal Extension

STRENGTHENS AND TONES: *Back muscles,*
Every muscle on the back of the body,
including muscles of the butt and thighs
STRETCHES: *Front side of the body*
IMPROVES: *Circulation to the spine, Enhances*
lymphatic system, Improves digestion

This pose improves spinal flexibility and relieves lower-back tension. In yoga, it is known to remove excess fat from around the liver. You will also be strengthening your hip joints, shoulders, and upper back.

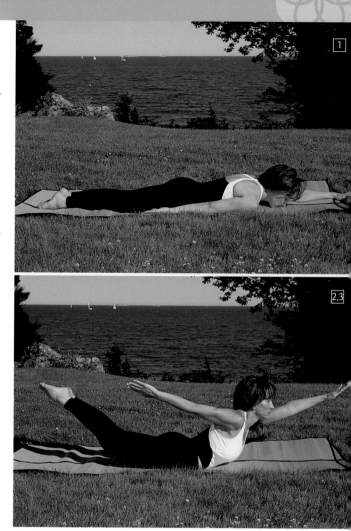

DIRECTIONS

1. Lie facedown on the floor with your left arm stretched out in front of you and your right arm stretched out behind you. Inhale.

2. Exhale, and lift and extend your arms, raising both legs back and away from your body, to a challenging height.

3. Hold the pose for 5 breaths, then release.

4. Repeat 3 times on this side.

5. Lower yourself toward the floor, switch arms, and repeat the pose.

NOTE: *If you need padding for your pelvis or hip bones, place a soft towel on your mat for extra cushioning.*

> **FLAB-FIGHTING FACT**
>
> This pose is great for improving muscle tone in the back, butt, and thighs.

Bow Pose

STRETCHES AND TONES: *Back muscles*

STRETCHES: *Front side of the body*

IMPROVES: *Spinal flexibility*

This is an intense backbend that stretches your entire spine and all the muscles along it. It is also a great chest opener and a profound release for the front of the shoulders, hips, and thighs.

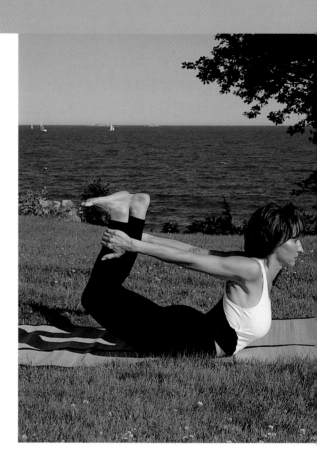

DIRECTIONS

1. Lie flat on your stomach. Bend your knees and keep them about hip-width apart.

2. Reach backward with your arms straight and grasp your ankles. Inhale.

3. Exhale while arching your entire body upward, pulling against your hands with your legs and raising your head, chest, and thighs off the floor. Hold for 5 breaths.

4. Lower your body slowly to the floor.

5. Repeat the pose twice.

FLAB-FIGHTING FACT

This pose helps in removing excess fat in your back and buttocks.

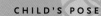

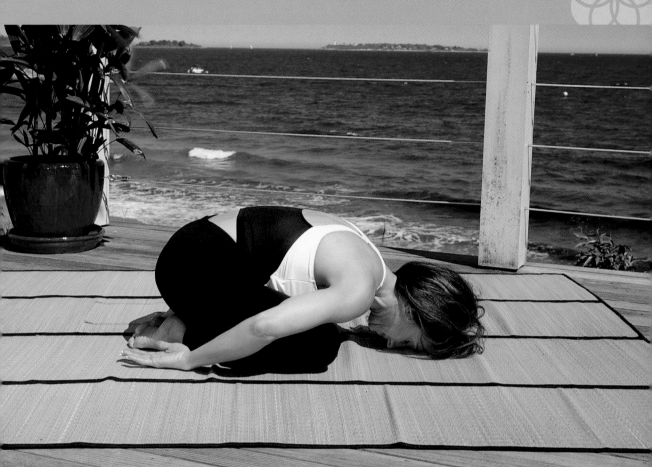

Child's Pose

Important: You need to follow these back exercises with the Child's Pose, which is a counterposture to the backbends, but do not put your arms forward.

DIRECTIONS

1 Kneel on the floor, bringing your buttocks toward your heels.

2 Place your arms lengthwise alongside your body.

3 Relax your neck muscles, bringing your forehead to the floor, rounding your spine and shoulders. Relax into the Child's Pose.

Bridge Pose

STRENGTHENS AND TONES: *Legs, thighs, hips, and abdomen; Neck and back muscles*

STRETCHES: *Neck and shoulders, Spine*

IMPROVES: *Spinal flexibility*

The Bridge Pose is incredible for toning the butt and thighs. It brings great flexibility to the spine and it stretches and strengthens neck and back muscles.

DIRECTIONS

1. Lie flat on your back, bending your knees and placing the soles of your feet on the floor. Your heels should touch your buttocks, or get as close as possible.

2. Turn your toes in slightly, making sure your feet and knees are slightly wider apart than your hips.

3. Raise and squeeze your thighs and buttocks, arching your back upward. Lift your hips high, raising your chest and navel as high as possible without moving your feet or shoulders. Keep those feet flat on the floor!

4. Bring your arms under your body, interlacing your fingers and straightening your arms flat on the floor, pressing them down. Hold this pose for 10 breaths.

5. Immediately prepare to go into the Extended Bridge Pose with One Leg Extended. Walk your right foot toward the middle of your mat.

6. Stay in the pose, bringing your arms alongside your body while lifting your left leg and extending your toes upward.

7. Flex your foot and bring it toward the floor.

8. Repeat pointed toes and flexed foot 5 times.

9. Return to the full Bridge Pose—knees bent, feet flat on the floor.

10. Repeat on the other side.

11. Return to the full Bridge Pose for 10 more breaths.

FLAB-FIGHTING FACT

The intense tightening of butt and thighs develops muscle and reduces fat.

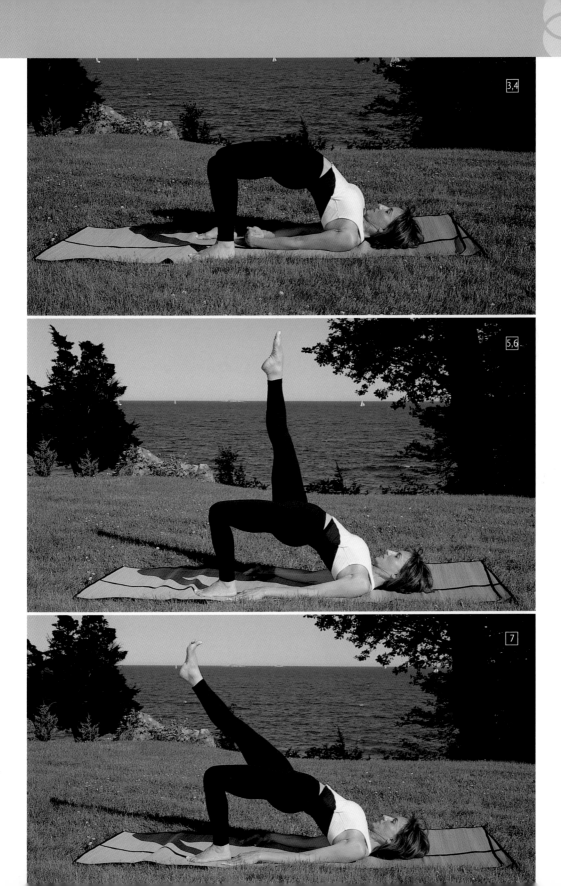

3,4

5,6

7

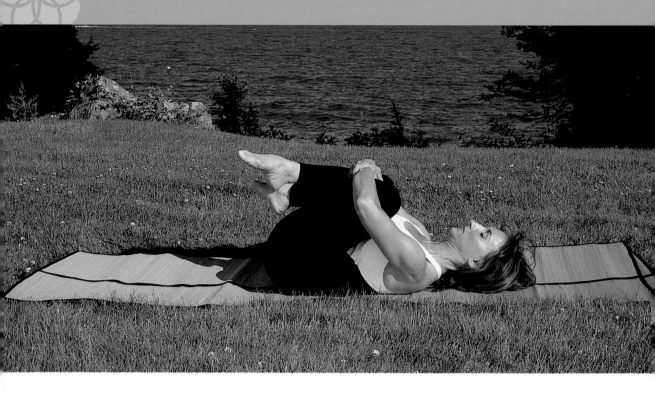

Knees to Chest Pose

STRETCHES AND TONES: *Lower back*

This pose is to be done immediately following the backbends. It releases and stretches the lower back.

DIRECTIONS

1 Bring both of your knees tight against your chest.

2 Wrap both arms around your knees in a hug, pulling them in close. Hold for a few breaths, or until you feel your spine and abs relax.

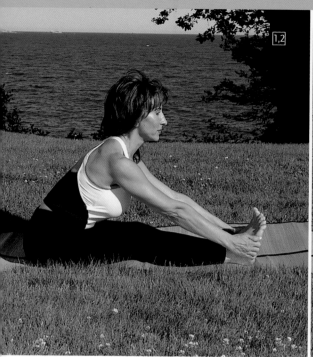

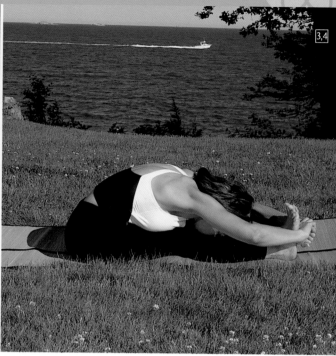

Seated Forward Bend

This pose will give you an intense stretch in the back of your body as you fold forward. It is a wonderful counterposture to all the backbends, and will leave you feeling balanced and restored.

DIRECTIONS

1 Sit with your legs stretched out in front of you, knees straight. Pull you toes back toward your body.

2 Lift your arms, elongating your spine and stretching your entire back up and forward.

3 Hinge at the hips and fall forward, grabbing your feet (or as far as you can reach—toes, ankles, heels, shins). Bring your chest down toward your thighs. It is important never to force the stretch.

4 Relax your shoulders and your neck, looking toward your legs. Hold this pose for 5 breaths.

Sun Salutation with Push-up

Repeat from pages 88–93, but add the following element:

DIRECTIONS

1. From the Sun Salutation in the Plank Position, transition to the Chaturanga Pose, pushing up and down 3 times for an extra challenge (see steps 6, 7A, 7B, below).

2. Continue with the Sun Salutation.

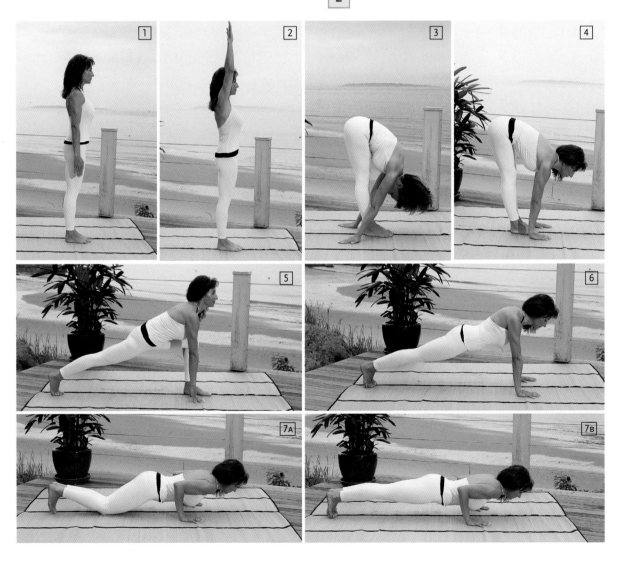

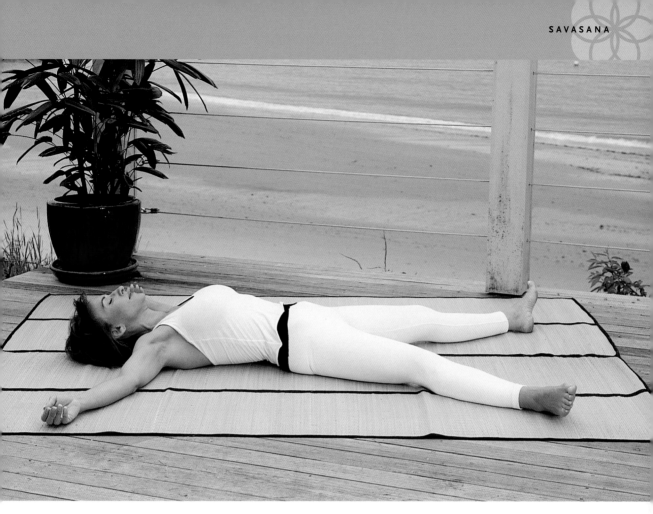

Savasana

DIRECTIONS

1. Lie flat on your back with your feet apart and your toes relaxed and facing out.

2. Place your arms out from your sides, with your palms up.

3. Close your eyes and consciously release and relax each and every muscle, transferring all the weight of your body to the floor.

4. Slowly bring your focus to your breath, and feel the rhythmic movement of your body as you breathe in and out. Really get in touch with your body and your breath, holding the pose for 5 to 10 minutes.

5. Wrap your arms around your knees, drawing them into your chest, and roll to your right side into a fetal position.

Day Five

Day Five is full of Abdominal Strengthening Poses. No muscle group causes more agony and concern than the abs. Everyone wants firm and flat abs, and this is absolutely possible through these simple but dynamic exercises. You will firm and strengthen the abs and replace fat with muscle. Strong abs in balance with a strong back will help you feel more powerful in your everyday life.

The rectus abdominus is the big flat muscle that runs between your ribcage and your pubic bone. It stabilizes your torso, and when it is toned, it looks terrific. The internal and external obliques wrap around the sides of the torso. When all these muscles are toned, you will have that washboard effect!

Sun Salutation

Repeat from pages 88–93.

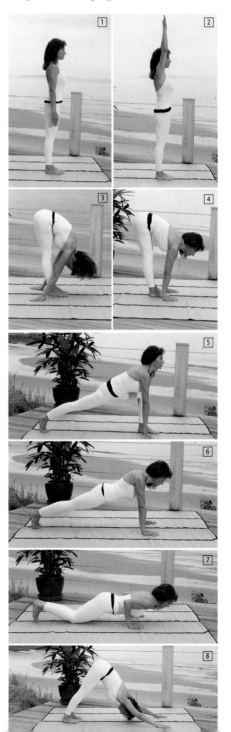

Boat Pose

STRENGTHENS: *Abdominal muscles, Hip flexors, Quads*

IMPROVES: *Abdominal muscle tone and builds body strength*

This pose strengthens and tones the frontal abdominal muscles as well as the abdominal obliques bilaterally, which also gives the lower back support internally.

DIRECTIONS

1 While seated, lift your feet off the floor and wrap your arms around your legs.

2 Contract your abdominal muscles as you lift your legs and torso up, bringing your arms out to the side.

3 Stay balanced on your sit bones and lift your ribcage. Ideally legs should be straight—if you have had a back injury or this is too advanced for you, bend your knees. You can also hold the backs of your thighs or knees. Hold for 10 breaths.

4 Repeat this pose 3 times.

CAUTION: *Beware of rounding or overarching your lower back. Lock those abdominal muscles to prevent this.*

FLAB-FIGHTING FACT
Muscle tone replaces fat, especially around the midsection of the body.

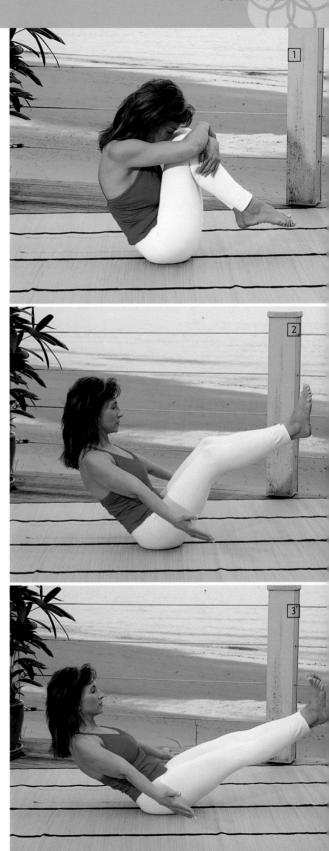

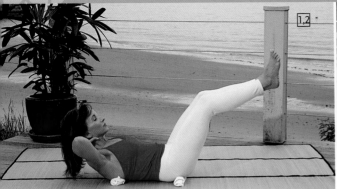

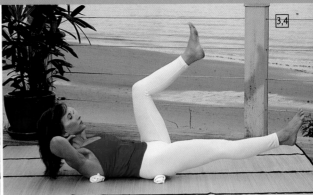

Abdominal 1

STRENGTHENS AND TONES: *Abdominals*

IMPROVES: *Overall strength and balance*

Perform all the abdominal exercises in good form—no sloppy movements. Awareness is your weapon. Be precise in your movement to become more efficient and effective. It is also important to connect the mind and body, and focus on the muscle you are working. All of these poses should be performed as one continuous exercise. In the Abdominal 1, 2, 3, and 4 poses, you can add an optional element by rolling two small, thin towels and placing one toward the top of your back, the other where your hips meet the floor. This helps to isolate the abdominal muscles.

FLAB-FIGHTING FACT

As you tone your abdominal muscles you will slim your waistline and replace fat with muscle.

DIRECTIONS

1. Lie on your back with your knees bent. Interlace your fingers behind your neck, placing your thumbs on either side of your neck to support your head.

2. Inhale while lifting your head off the floor, supporting your head with your hands and keeping your elbows out to the sides. Lift your shoulders off the floor to engage your abdominal muscles.

3. Tighten and pull your lower abdominals in as you lift your legs in a bent position.

4. Exhale while lowering your right leg toward the floor. Flex your foot and straighten your leg, keeping your spine absolutely flat on the floor, and make sure your abs are not bulging out as you lower your leg as far as you can while maintaining proper position. If your spine starts to overarch, do not lower your legs as far.

5. Lift your leg straight up and down, repeating 10 times.

6. Repeat with the opposite leg.

7. Return to the starting position, and immediately begin Abdominal 2.

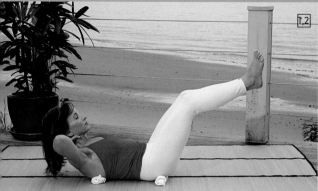 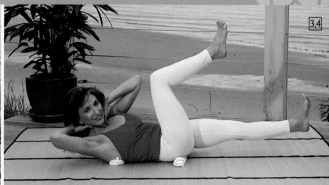

Abdominal 2

This pose engages the oblique (side) abdominal muscles, as well as the rectus abdominus (frontal) muscle, which helps shape your waist. The key to toning the obliques is in the twisting of the torso.

DIRECTIONS

1. Lie on your back with your knees bent. Interlace your fingers behind your neck, placing your thumbs on either side of your neck to support your head.

2. Inhale while lifting your head and shoulder blades off the floor, keeping your elbows out to the sides and supporting your head so as to engage your upper abs. Lift your shoulders off the floor to engage your abdominal muscles.

3. Tighten and pull your lower abs in as you lift your legs, bent at a 90-degree angle.

4. Exhale, keeping your back flat on the floor while extending your left elbow toward your right knee. Keep your elbows open and your lower abs pulled in tight toward your back.

5. Inhale, change legs, and exhale to the other side. Repeat 10 to 20 times at a brisk pace.

6. Return to the Knees to Chest Pose, and immediately begin Abdominal 3.

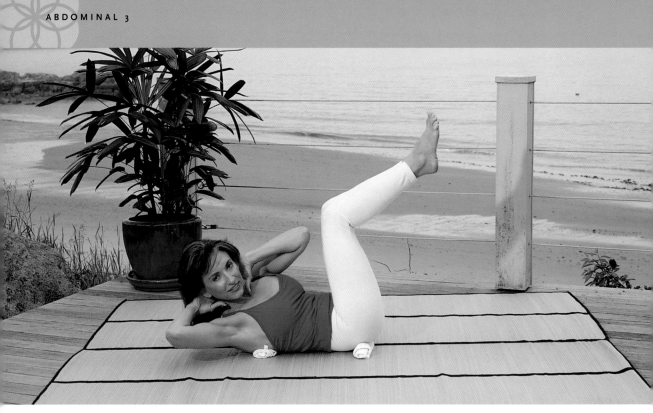

Abdominal 3

This pose engages all frontal and oblique muscles.

DIRECTIONS

1 Lie on your back with your knees bent. Interlace your fingers behind your neck, keeping your elbows open to support your neck, and keep your head off the floor. (This works the upper abdominals.)

2 Pull your abdominal muscles in toward your back as you bring your knees toward your chest. This is the most vital part toward performing the exercise correctly. Extend your knees slightly, working your lower abs.

3 Inhale as you pull your abdominals toward your back. Consciously feel your back flatten into the floor. If at any moment you arch your spine, you immediately put stress on your lower back and will not get the maximum benefits of this exercise. Maintain a flat back throughout.

4 Exhale while lifting your shoulder blades off the floor as you crunch, twisting your torso, bringing your left shoulder toward your right knee, working the entire abdominal region and obliques. The range of movement is small, and you should move slowly.

5 Lift and lower your shoulder blades, twisting to the side, 10 times each side. Release your abdominals and bring both your knees in toward your chest.

MODIFICATION

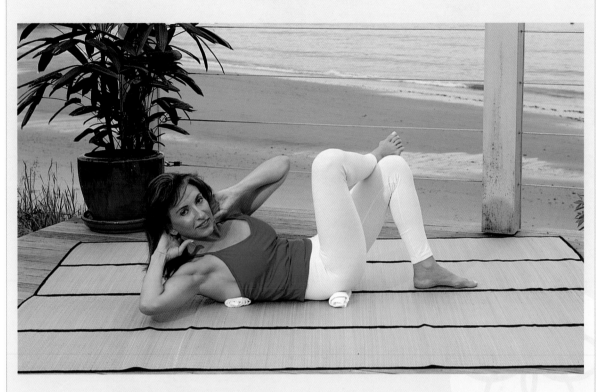

You can modify this pose by placing your left foot on the floor, and your right ankle on your left knee, then twisting your left shoulder toward your right knee.

1 Bring your right knee in toward your chest as close as you can.

2 Interlace your fingers around your knee in a hug, and hold for a few breaths or until you feel your spine and abs relax.

3 Repeat with the other leg.

4 Go directly into Abdominal 4.

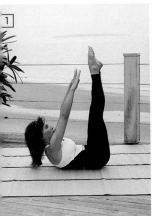 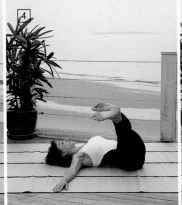 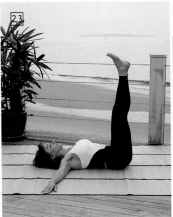 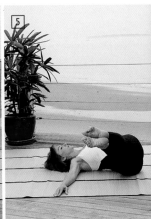

Abdominal 4

DIRECTIONS

1   Lie on your back and reach your hands to your toes—hold for 5 breaths.

2   Bring your upper torso back to the floor.

3   Inhale, straighten your legs to 90 degrees, and bring your arms out to the side, keeping your knees and ankles together and your upper torso flat on the floor.

4   Exhale, slowly lowering your legs halfway down to the floor to the right of you. Hold for 5 breaths.

5   Lower until you are a few inches off the floor. Hold for 5 breaths.

6   Inhale and lift back to the center. Repeat on the other side.

MODIFICATION

You can modify this pose by bending your knees.

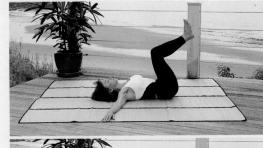

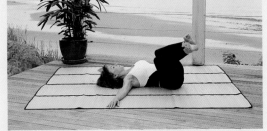

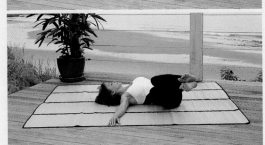

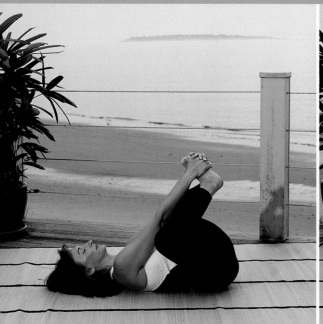
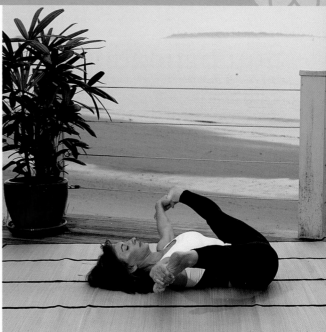

Abdominal Release and Stretch

DIRECTIONS

1 While still lying on the floor, bring the soles of your feet together. This will release your abdominals, and release your spine.

2 Holding the inside of your feet or your thighs (wherever you can reach), bring your legs out to the side for a stretch to the inner and outer thighs, releasing the abdominals and spine.

Sun Salutation

Repeat from pages 88–93.

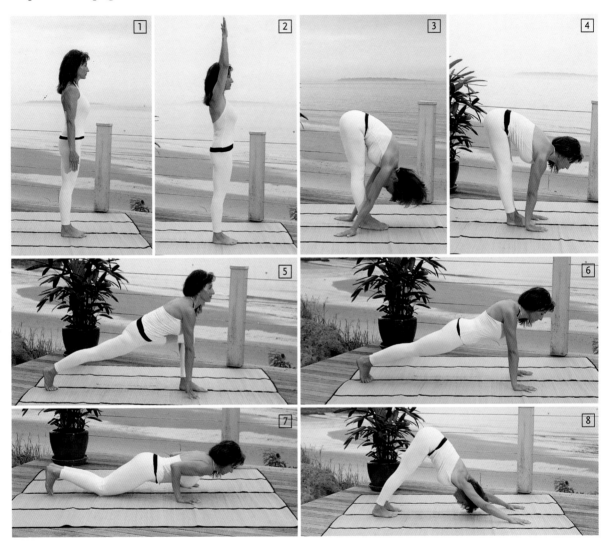

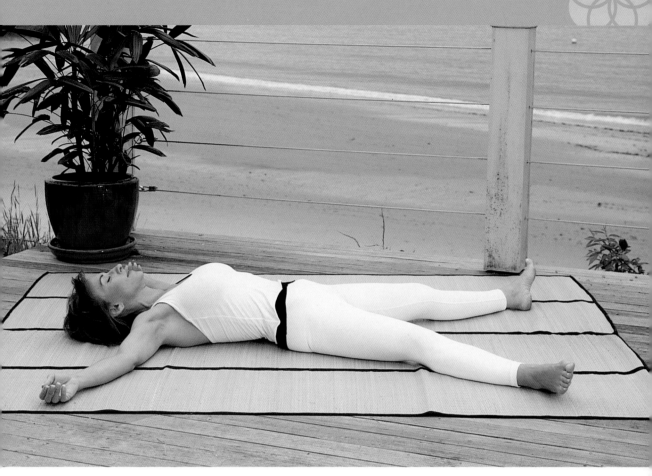

Savasana

DIRECTIONS

1 Lie flat on your back with your feet apart and your toes relaxed and facing out.

2 Place your arms out from your sides, with your palms up.

3 Close your eyes and consciously release and relax each and every muscle, transferring all the weight of your body to the floor.

4 Slowly bring your focus to your breath, and feel the rhythmic movement of your body as you breathe in and out. Really get in touch with your body and your breath, holding the pose for 5 to 10 minutes.

5 Wrap your arms around your knees, drawing them into your chest, and roll to your right side into a fetal position.

Day Six

For this day, we will concentrate on the Sculpting and Toning Upper Body Poses. These postures are particularly useful for the shoulders, arms, and back, building strength and flexibility in these areas. These various poses are dynamic in getting rid of upper-body flab!

Sun Salutation

Repeat from pages 88–93.

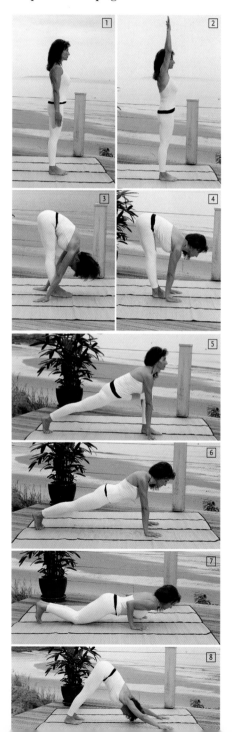

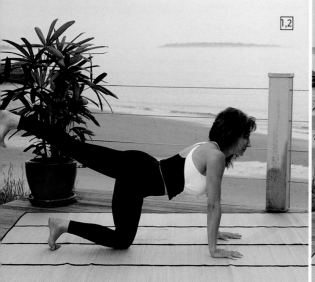

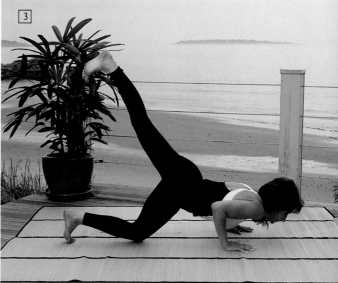

Active Cat with Yoga Press

STRENGTHENS AND TONES: *Muscles of the upper arms and back, Triceps; Conditions the abdominals*

IMPROVES: *Upper-body strength*

This is an empowering pose that will strengthen your upper arms and back, and tone your triceps.

DIRECTIONS

1. Kneel on your hands and knees.

2. Inhale while lifting your left leg straight up behind you, as high as you can without overarching your back.

3. Exhale, and bring your body forward by bending your elbows into a push-up position, tucking them in and holding your ribcage, keeping your body firm and supported.

4. Inhale, and push away from the floor, back to starting position.

5. Repeat 5 times.

6. Now, repeat with your right leg

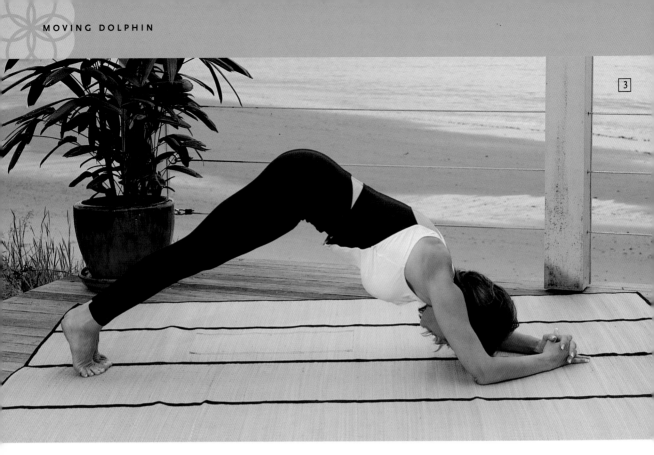

Moving Dolphin

STRENGTHENS AND TONES: *Upper body, particularly shoulders*

STRETCHES: *Stretches and improves flexibility in the shoulders*

IMPROVES: *Alignment of the upper back and shoulder girdle*

The Dolphin is one of the best postures for developing strength and flexibility in your shoulders and improving alignment of your upper back and shoulder girdle. You will build tremendous strength, and at the same time reshape and tone your upper body.

DIRECTIONS

1. Start on your hands and knees.

2. Lower your forearms to the floor, elbows under your shoulders, and interlace your fingers.

3. Inhale, straighten your legs, and lift your pelvis, elevating the sit bones.

4. Exhale while shifting your weight forward—your chest moves forward toward the floor between your forearms.

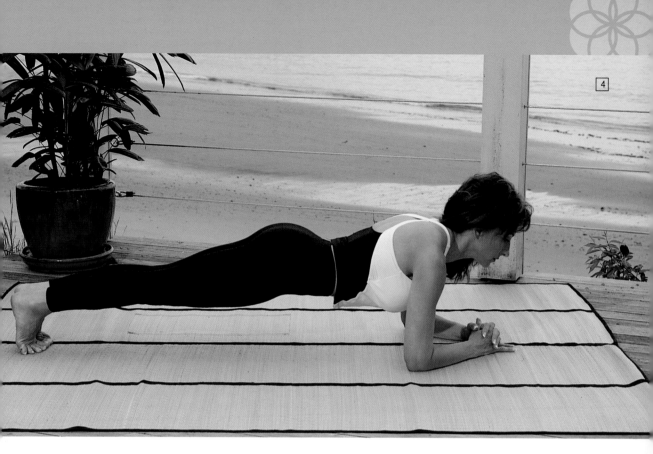

4

5 Inhale, and shift your weight back,
moving the chest behind the arms toward
the thighs.

6 Repeat 5 times.

7 End by coming back onto all fours.

8 Stretch back into the Child's Pose.

FLAB-FIGHTING FACT

This pose will reshape the upper body,
getting rid of excess flab, and will also
engage the abdominals.

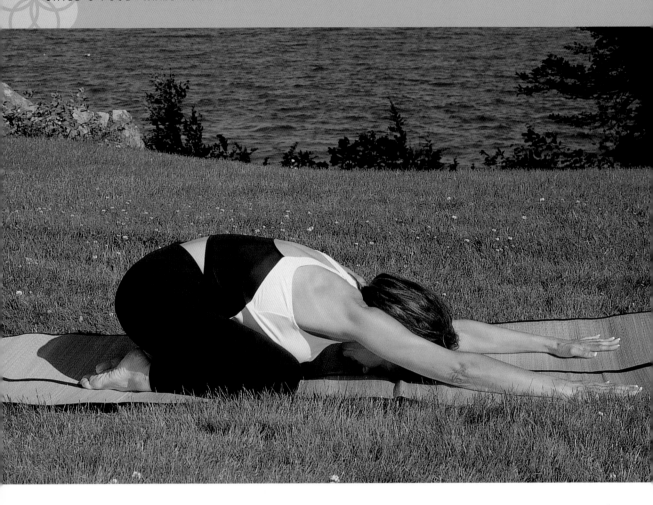

Child's Pose— Arms Forward

STRETCHES: *Spine and thigh muscles*
IMPROVES: *Circulation*

The Child's Pose reduces fatigue and tension and relaxes your lower back and neck. It slows down the heart rate and calms emotions.

DIRECTIONS

1. Kneel on the floor and bring your buttocks toward your heels.

2. Stretch your arms out in front of you.

3. Stretch your chin forward to the floor, rounding your spine and shoulders.

4. Relax your neck muscles, walking your fingers forward to get a stretch to the shoulders, and relax into the pose. Hold this pose for 3 breaths.

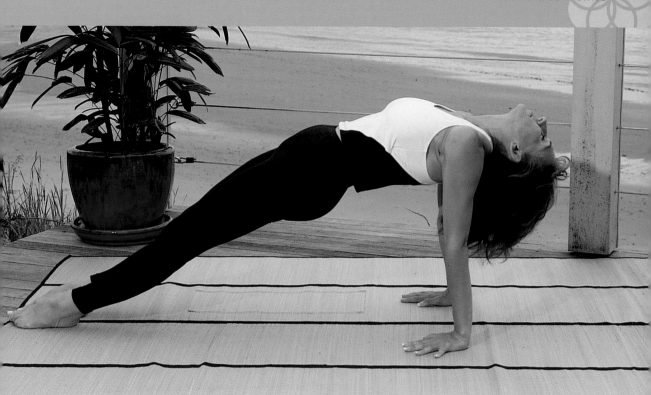

Inclined Plane

STRENGTHENS AND TONES: *Muscles in front of the shoulders, Biceps*

STRETCHES: *Front of the body*

IMPROVES: *Improves and tones the lumbar region*

This pose strengthens the whole body and tones the lumbar region of the spine and Achilles tendons. It also stretches and tones the muscles in the front of the shoulders and biceps.

FLAB-FIGHTING FACT

Muscle will replace flab—even hard-to-hit areas like the muscles in front of the shoulders.

DIRECTIONS

1. Sit with your legs stretched out in front of you.

2. Place the palms of your hands on the floor on either side of your body, just behind your buttocks, fingers facing forward.

3. Raise your buttocks and lift your body upward, pushing your hips up and making your body as straight as possible— you are trying to look like an inclined plane, remember!

4. Let you head hang back and down gently, keeping the soles of your feet flat on the floor and your arms and legs straight. Hold this pose for 5 breaths.

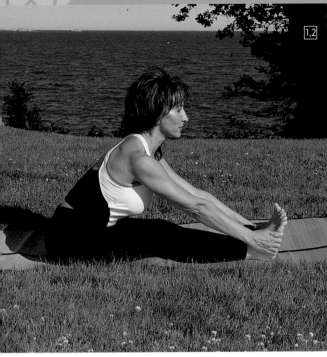 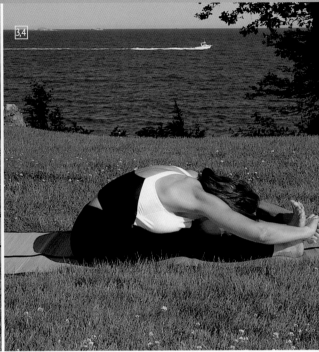

Seated Forward Bend

DIRECTIONS

1 Sit with your legs stretched out in front of you, knees straight. Pull your toes back toward your body.

2 Lift your arms, elongating your spine and stretching your entire back up and forward.

3 Hinge at the hips and fall forward, grabbing your feet (or as far as you can reach—toes, ankles, heels, shins). Bring your chest down toward your thighs. It is important never to force the stretch.

4 Relax your shoulders and your neck, looking toward your legs. Hold this pose for 5 breaths.

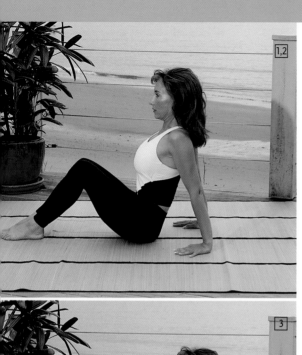

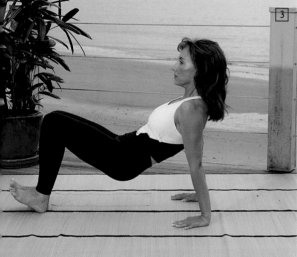

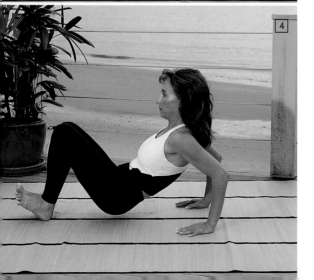

Sitting Triceps

STRENGTHENS AND TONES: *Triceps*

IMPROVES: *Overall body strength*

DIRECTIONS

1 Come into a seated position.

2 Inhale, placing your hands directly in line with your shoulders, with your arms bent, fingers facing forward.

3 Exhale, straightening your arms, and lift your torso off the floor.

4 Inhale, lowering your hips toward the floor with bent arms. Concentrate on using your triceps.

5 Repeat these tricep dips 10 times.

FLAB-FIGHTING FACT

Wave good-bye to waving triceps.

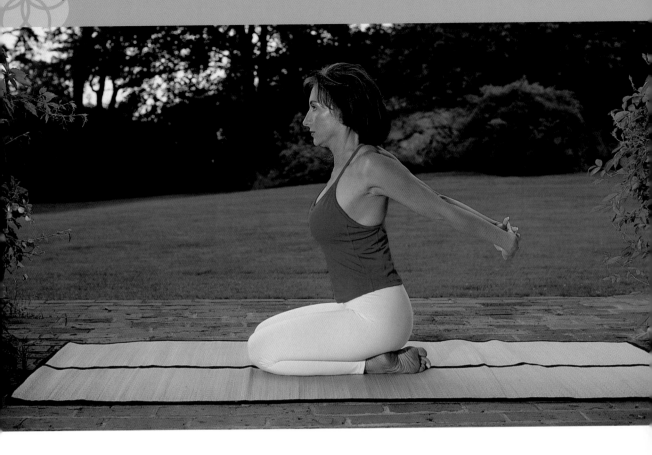

Arm, Shoulder, and Triceps Stretch

STRETCHES: *Arms, shoulders, and triceps*

DIRECTIONS

1 Kneel on the floor with your spine straight and interlace your fingers behind your back.

2 With your shoulders pushed back and your arms straight, lift your arms as high as you can, feeling a good stretch in your arms and shoulders. Hold this pose for 5 breaths.

Sun Salutation

Repeat from pages 88–93.

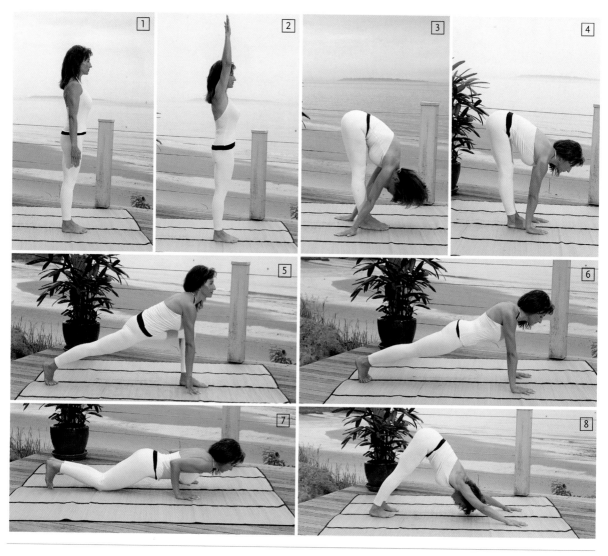

Savasana

Repeat from page 40.

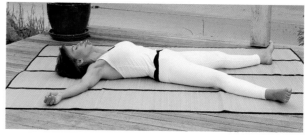

7 Day Seven

Day Seven is devoted to Lower Body Sculpting Poses—in short, getting the flab out of your butt! These poses isometrically sculpt your buttocks, thighs, and back muscles. In the Prayer Twist, like all Twisting Poses, all the internal organs get massaged. It is a powerful way to detoxify organs and glands, which boosts your overall health.

Sun Salutation

Repeat from pages 88–93.

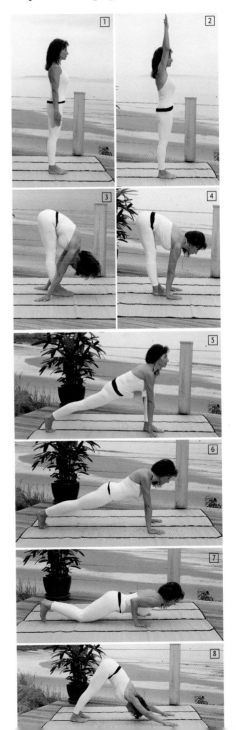

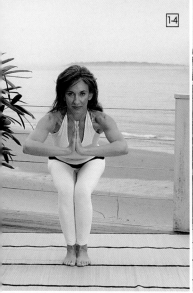
1-4

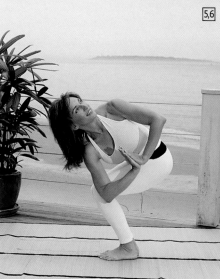
5,6

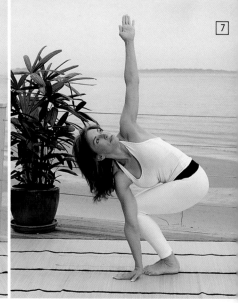
7

Squatted Prayer Twist

STRENGTHENS AND TONES: *Buttocks, thighs, and back muscles*

STRETCHES: *Spine and muscles of the back*

IMPROVES: *Strength in the mid- and lower back*

DIRECTIONS

1 From a standing position dip your hips low.

2 Squeeze your knees level and together.

3 Press your buttocks back and pull your chest forward.

4 Bring your hands together in prayer position.

5 Twist from your torso, not from your arms.

6 Place your right elbow on the outside of your left knee, stacking your upper shoulder over your lower shoulder. Hold for 5 breaths.

7 Extend your arms out. Hold for 5 breaths.

8 Bring your hands back to prayer position for 5 breaths.

9 Release into a standing position.

FLAB-FIGHTING FACT

You will sculpt your buttocks and thighs, replacing fat with muscle. Like all twisting poses, prayer twist is a powerful way to detoxify organs and glands by massaging those areas. You will also be boosting your overall health.

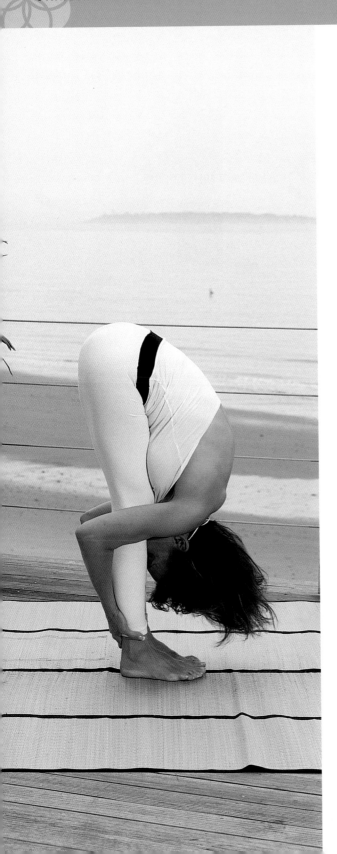

Standing Forward Bend

STRENGTHENS AND TONES: *Back*

STRETCHES: *Hamstrings, Back—opens every vertebra in the spine*

IMPROVES: *Flexibility throughout the body*

DIRECTIONS

1. From the Squatted Prayer Position (with your right foot forward), straighten both legs.

2. Bring your arms out to your sides, and pull your hands toward your heart center, standing upright.

3. Inhale, lifting your arms over your head.

4. Exhale, folding your body forward from the hips (not from the middle of the back), keeping your spine straight. Relax your hip joints so that your body bends without your spine curving. Place your hands on the floor next to your feet; if you cannot do that, start out by grabbing hold of your shins or ankles.

5. Lift your buttocks and lower your head to your shins. Relax your abdominal muscles, easing into the pose. (Don't force it.) Hold for 5 breaths.

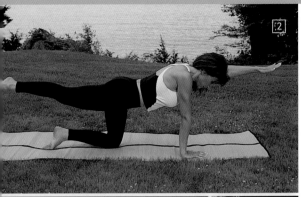

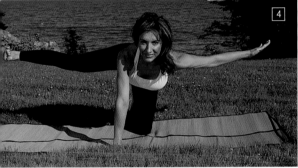

Spinal Balancing and Hip Rotation

STRENGTHENS AND TONES: *Thighs, Shoulders, Upper back*

STRETCHES: *Spine; Flexes hips*

IMPROVES: *Balance*

The Spinal Balancing Pose is great for improving balance and lengthening your spine, and as we continue into Hip Rotation Pose, you will tone and sculpt those thigh and butt muscles. This targets the areas where most exercises do not reach to lessen the fat. This pose is also great for opening your pelvis for improved flexibility.

DIRECTIONS

1. Begin this pose on all fours, knees directly below your hips, hands directly below your shoulders.

2. Extend your left arm forward and your right leg back, holding them parallel to the floor. Stretch your spine from your fingertips to your toes, using all your strength. Feel the energy extend from the center of your body in both directions.

3. Gaze down at the floor, being careful not to lift your head. Hold this pose for 5 breaths.

4. Extend your left arm out to the side at shoulder level and your right leg out to the side at hip level. Hold this pose for 10 breaths.

5. Repeat one more time with the same arm and leg.

6. Repeat steps 1–5 again, but use the alternate arms and legs to complete the exercise.

FLAB-FIGHTING FACT
This pose flattens the stomach and improves overall strength and muscle gain by toning the thighs and buttocks muscles.

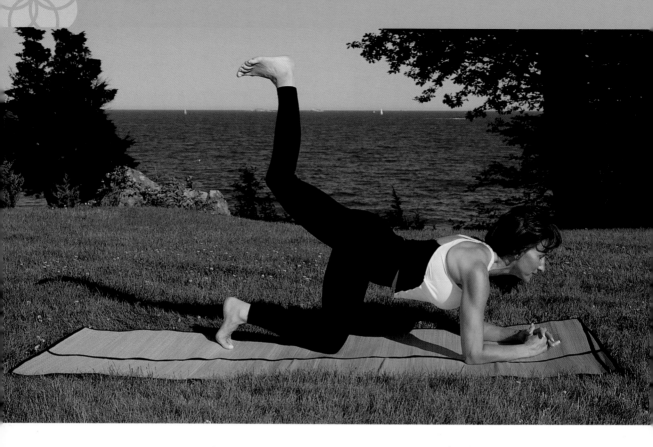

Buttocks Firmer 1

STRENGTHENS AND TONES: *Thigh and buttocks muscles*

IMPROVES: Flexibility in the hips

This exercise, as with the abdominals, is a series of poses that tackle the difficult area of the buttocks, where flab often gathers. Well, not anymore!

DIRECTIONS

1. Get into the all-fours position.

2. Inhale, bringing your left leg up behind your body and bending it at the knee.

3. Exhale, pressing your left foot toward the ceiling, and pulse.

4. Repeat 5 sets of 10 pulses.

5. Repeat on the other side.

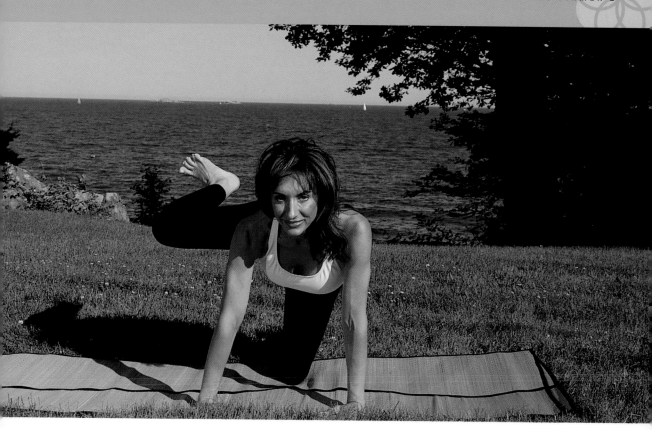

Buttocks Firmer 2

DIRECTIONS

1. Get into the all-fours position. Inhale.

2. Exhale, lifting your right leg, bent at the knee, from your hip joint to the side.

3. Repeat 3 sets of 10.

4. Switch sides and repeat.

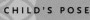

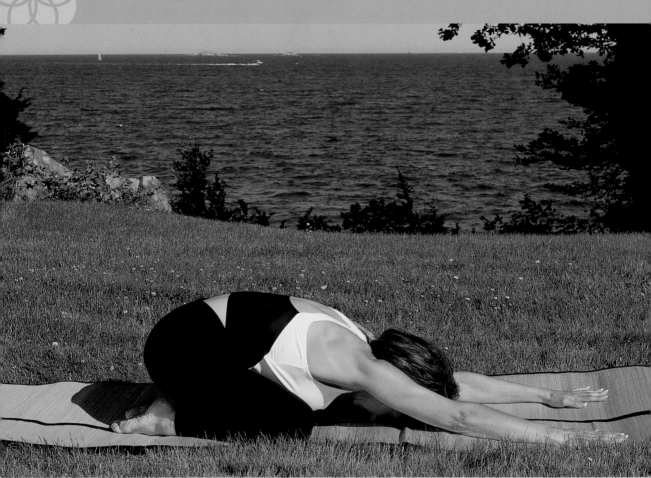

Child's Pose—
Arms Forward

STRETCHES: *Spine and thigh muscles*
IMPROVES: *Circulation*

The Child's Pose reduces fatigue and tension and relaxes your lower back and neck. It slows down the heart rate and calms emotions.

DIRECTIONS

1   Kneel on the floor and bring your buttocks toward your heels.

2   Stretch your arms out in front of you.

3   Stretch your chin forward to the floor, rounding your spine and shoulders.

4   Relax your neck muscles, walking your fingers forward to get a stretch to the shoulders, and relax into the pose. Hold this pose for 3 breaths.

Sun Salutation

Repeat from pages 88–93.

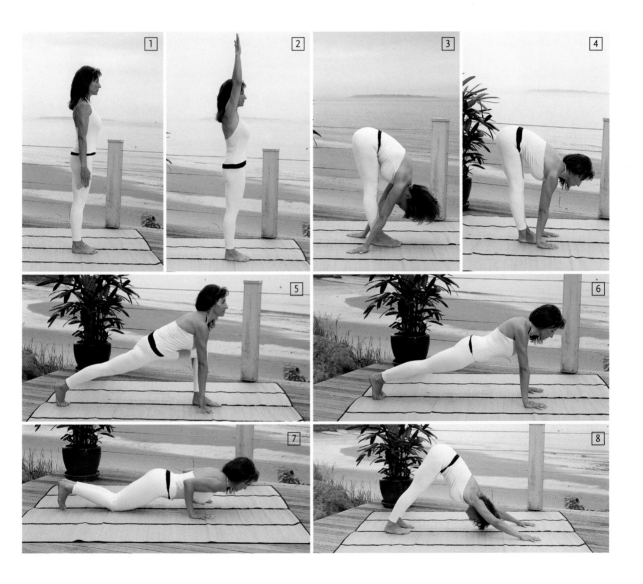

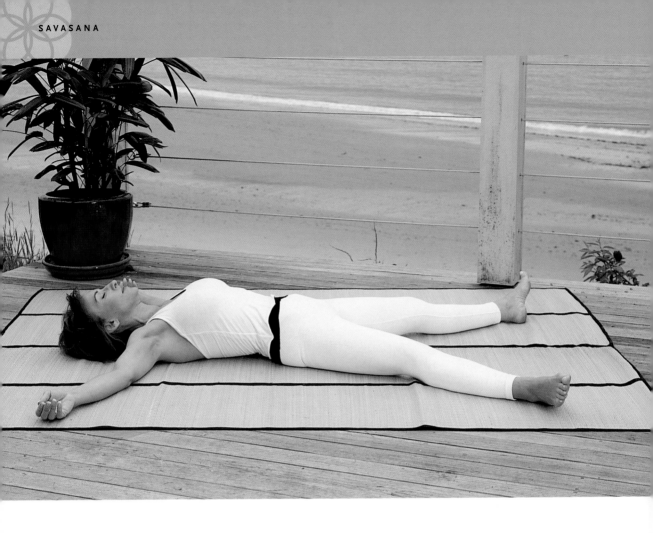

Savasana

DIRECTIONS

1　Lie flat on your back with your feet apart and your toes relaxed and facing out.

2　Place your arms out from your sides, with your palms up.

3　Close your eyes and consciously release and relax each and every muscle, transferring all the weight of your body to the floor.

4　Slowly bring your focus to your breath, and feel the rhythmic movement of your body as you breathe in and out. Really get in touch with your body and your breath, holding the pose for 5 to 10 minutes.

5　Wrap your arms around your knees, drawing them into your chest, and roll to your right side into a fetal position.

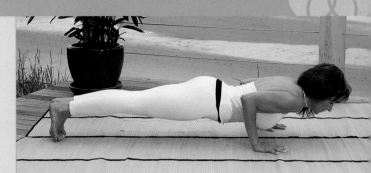

Day Eight

Repeat Day One, but replace the Modified Chaturanga with the Challenge Chaturanga.

Challenge Chaturanga

DIRECTIONS

1. Once you have mastered the Modified Chaturanga Pose, test yourself further with this pose. Remain in the Plank Pose, keeping your knees off the floor.

2. Bend your elbows without bending your knees. Keep your arms tight against your ribcage. Keep your body firm and supported, and don't let it sag. It if does, rest your knees on the floor in the Modified Chaturanga Pose and continue from there.

3. While keeping your palms flat on the floor, lengthen your spine and keep your thighs active as you tighten your tummy muscles and gaze at the floor. Hold this pose for 5 breaths.

4. If this is still too much of a challenge, hold off until you can do it. In any event, add an additional Sun Salutation at the beginning and end of your routine. These additional Sun Salutations will become your new baseline.

Day 9 | *Repeat Day Two with the extra Sun Salutations.*

Day 10 | *Repeat Day Three with the extra Sun Salutations.*

Day 11 | *Repeat Day Four with the extra Sun Salutations.*

Day 12 | *Repeat Day Five with the extra Sun Salutations.*

Day 13 | *Repeat Day Six with the extra Sun Salutations.*

Day 14 | *Repeat Day Seven with the extra Sun Salutations.*

Day 15 | *This is your first day off in two weeks—enjoy it!*

Day 16 | *Now it's time to get back to your routine. This time, repeat Day One with the extra Sun Salutations, but increase the difficulty by adding an additional five breaths to every pose that asks for them—thus, "hold for 5 breaths" becomes "hold for 10 breaths"! Sound intense? Don't worry—you can do it!*

Day 17 | *Repeat Day Two with the extra Sun Salutations and the additional five breaths.*

Day 18 | *Repeat Day Three with the extra Sun Salutations and the additional five breaths.*

Day 19 | *Repeat Day Four with the extra Sun Salutations and the additional five breaths.*

Day 20 | *Repeat Day Five with the extra Sun Salutations and the additional five breaths.*

Day 21 | *Repeat Day Six with the extra Sun Salutations and the additional five breaths.*

Day 22 | *Repeat Day Seven with the extra Sun Salutations and the additional five breaths.*

Day 23 | *You've earned a second day off!*

Day 24 | *Repeat Day One with the extra Sun Salutations and the additional five breaths.*

Day 25 | *Repeat Day Two with the extra Sun Salutations and the additional five breaths.*

Day 26 | *Repeat Day Three with the extra Sun Salutations and the additional five breaths. Add more of a challenge to the Standing Head to Knee (One Leg) Pose by interlacing your fingers behind your back. (See page 120.) Then bring your arms toward your shoulders as high as possible to get a good stretch.*

Day 27 | *Repeat Day Four with the extra Sun Salutations and the additional five breaths.*

Day 28 | *Repeat Day Five with the extra Sun Salutations and the additional five breaths. Add more of a challenge to the Boat Pose by keeping your legs straight rather than bending them and/or holding them with your arms.*

Day 29 | *Repeat Day Six with the extra Sun Salutations and the additional five breaths.*

Day 30 | *Repeat Day Seven with the extra Sun Salutations and the additional five breaths.*

You have now completed your Total 30-Day Flab-Burning Program! From here on out, you should need to do only maintenance—three times a week—to keep off the flab. But more importantly, you have begun to achieve overall body health.

CHAPTER 6

Knowing Success Is Yours

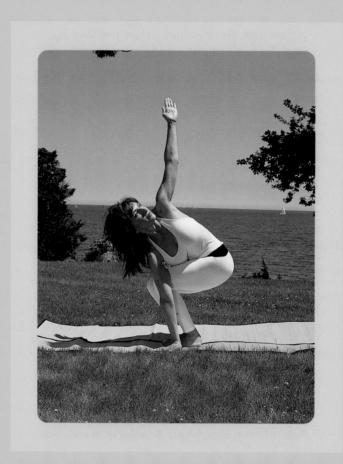

B elieve it or not, you are now ready to go out on your own. When you first looked at this book and read the words "Yoga Fights Flab," you may have questioned it, expecting the same pitfalls as in many of the programs you may have tried. By now you should realize that this program is different. It is possible to be lean, fit, healthy, and centered. As a result, you will never see yourself as trapped in your same old boundaries.

MAINTAINING YOUR NEW FIGURE

While a commitment to exercise is a wonderful thing, maintaining it usually requires some inspiration. I hope that my book can inspire you like it has so many of my students. To keep you going, here are some truly encouraging Stories. Namaste!

Randi Schwartz

42 years old, sales management

I walked into Glenda's yoga class two years ago upon recommendation from a co-worker who found her class to be the most challenging yet effective class she had ever taken. After years of battling the bulge, trying every diet imaginable and subjecting myself to grueling workouts with various trainers that only made my body get bigger, I finally found the workout that would prove to be the answer to my prayers. I participate in Glenda's class three times a week and I have not only lost thirty-eight pounds, but have also completely reshaped my entire body. My arms and shoulders have shape and my legs are not only trimmer but actually have less cellulite and incredible definition. My stomach is flatter and I can wear clothes that are more body conscious and flattering. I feel I have peeled off a layer of fat and am a shadow of my former bulky self. I now have renewed confidence, enjoy going shopping for new clothes, and have energy galore. When someone compliments me and asks me how I changed my body, I tell them to experience Glenda's class and they will never have to worry about fighting fat again.

Andy Jent

34 years old, senior director of management consulting

Last year, close to my thirty-fourth birthday, I made a decision to get back in shape. My plan included eating right and working out regularly, which I had not done seriously since high school. I had been running and attending spin classes at least once or twice a week, but it did not seem to be doing the trick. I attended one of Glenda's classes and found it to be an incredibly good workout and stress reliever. My wife had been a big proponent of Glenda's class and convinced me that I would really enjoy it. The first several times that I attended the class I felt awkward and *very* out of shape. However, having been a wrestler in high school, this was the first workout that I had done since then that came anywhere close to the feeling that I had during wrestling practice. It combined the elements of stretching, weight lifting, and a lot of sweating into a one-hour-and-fifteen-minute workout. There is no other workout that comes close to Glenda's classes. Because my job forces me to travel regularly, I am able to attend Glenda's classes only once or twice a week. I still run while I am on the road and spin on most Saturdays. The result thus far (over a three-month period) is that I have lost twenty-five pounds, three inches off my waist, and I have a lot more energy than I have had in a long time. I am convinced that the yoga portion of my workout is the biggest contributor to both my slimming and my weight loss. I had a goal to lose forty pounds when I started, and with only fifteen to go, I am sure that with my continued attendance at yoga I will get there very soon. Thanks, Glenda, for your support.

Erin Braxton

29 years old, advertising executive

Glenda's yoga class has been the best thing I've ever done. First of all, it is the first time that I've actually enjoyed working out. No matter what it takes, I will always make it to yoga class. Even if I have to leave work and come back later, I rarely miss. When I began taking Glenda's class almost two years ago, I thought it was one of the most challenging workouts I had ever had. But with Glenda as my model, I was determined to keep coming and to truly grasp the practice. At that time my body was at its worst. I had about twenty extra pounds that I wanted to shed, and I was soft. I had been trying to jog and do other cardio at the gym and weight lifting, but I never really enjoyed it and I wasn't seeing the results. Within a few weeks of beginning yoga, I began seeing results. My arm muscles became more defined and my upper-body strength even amazes me. The extra weight just started to come off. I now have a leaner build. Even though I've lost weight exercising in the past, this time it is more noticeable because my body is re-sculpted. I've encouraged numerous friends to come with me and many are now regulars.

Pam Brock

47 years old, homemaker/PTA president

Exercise has always been an important part of my daily life. Not only am I interested in the physical appearance that is obtained through exercise, but more importantly, the health benefits. Through the years I have done combinations of exercises to try and get the results I wanted, but not until I was introduced to Glenda's unique yoga class was I able to get the results—plus more—in just one class. Not only have the benefits I received from her class sculpted my body and made it firm, strong, and flexible, but the mind/body benefits of her class have improved my life. I am forty-seven, and people are always amazed when I tell them how old I am. I know Glenda's yoga program has given me a more youthful feeling inside and out. At my age the strength I have gotten from Glenda's guidance will carry me not only through the next weeks, months, years—but decades.

Finally, let me offer a comment from Vera Twining, who is perhaps my favorite success story, for obvious reasons.

Vera Twining

Glenda became a member of the Twining family a couple of years ago and her inspiration has changed my life in many wonderful ways. I have been an asthmatic for my entire adult life. Because of asthma, I was restricted in the amount of exercise activity I could endure.

Listening to Glenda share her thoughts about nutrition and yoga inspired me to become an active participant in yoga. Therefore, I joined the yoga club in Sun City West, Arizona, and for the past two winters I have looked forward to my early-morning yoga class. At our home in northern Michigan I enjoy starting my day by following the routine in Glenda's book *Yoga Turns Back the Clock*, which has proved to be beneficial to my health.

Recently, when I saw my pulmonary doctor he was amazed at how well I looked and was doing, and suggested whatever it was, I should continue with the program. I shared with my doctor that my daughter-in-law, Glenda, had inspired me to do yoga. He was impressed and confirmed yoga could be a beneficial part of my daily exercise.

Although asthma is still part of my life, I have found a yoga program that works for me. I have lost weight, toned my body, have more energy, improved breathing, and I feel good. Thanks, Glenda, for encouraging me to do yoga at my own pace. I am a true believer that yoga works wonders.

Afterword

It seems that parents can never stop worrying about their children, even when they are full-grown adults. I have two wonderful, adoring parents, now in their eighties and still living in South Africa, who have fretted over me since my divorce seven years ago. How could I, a woman living alone in America, make a future for myself? What career opportunities are there for women in their forties? And what about finding a loving and devoted husband to spend the rest of my life with?

My parents weren't the only ones who were worried. I had many goals in my younger days, graduating from high school at sixteen with my eye toward a career in medicine, or perhaps as a classical concert pianist (a pastime I continued throughout my teens). But in South Africa in the 1960s, women were expected to get married and have kids, not become professionals.

My mid-forties were other people's teenaged years. I already had a degree in fitness that I used only part time while serving as devoted mother and wife. After my divorce, I needed to earn a living, and fitness seemed like the best place to start. Becoming fit is not the easiest thing to do for anyone, not to mention a middle-aged housewife. But I dove right in, starting a program for overweight women and, later, founding a training group for men who needed to get physically fit to climb mountains—two classes of students at polar opposites.

I hurried to get all the degrees and certifications I could to teach fitness. And at the same time, I stumbled into yoga.

Despite no business training and some rusty skills, I refused to be put down. I studied for many grueling months, hours a day, with two Swamis in South Africa and wonderful teachers in America. I even helped run two yoga boot camps in the Yucatan, seventy people at each camp—invaluable experience in preparing me to get my program together.

Because I came to yoga having first learned many lessons from other exercise disciplines, my approach is not what you would find on a trip to India. I have taken traditional yoga to a new and energizing level where it not only refreshes and revitalizes the body, but actually burns off flab. It has the advantages of traditional yoga in that it is low impact and embraces an entire life philosophy, but it also works areas of the body often ignored by yoga, especially the abdominal muscles.

I started to incorporate yoga into my fitness regimen, combining yoga poses with strength-building poses where you work the upper body as much as the lower, incorporating strength-building abdominal exercises that are not only healthy but efficient. I incorporate traditional yoga poses with fitness to promote a well-rounded, whole personal health. And that's when my yoga career quickly took off.

At fifty-two, I am my own best testimonial—I practice every class with my students and have suffered no injuries even though I test myself to the limits. I am strong, flexible, toned, focused, calm, and hormonally balanced. I was always petite, but I never had toned or well-defined muscles. I have replaced fat with muscle and my body has become totally toned and supple. My friends and clients continue to be amazed by my youthful appearance.

My classes are jam-packed—reservations are almost always needed for every class—and all of this has happened in the past three years. For me, reaching these students of all ages has energized me in every sphere of my life.

I have a tighter body now than I ever dreamed possible. My body-fat ratio is 15 percent—incredible for a menopausal woman—and all since I started teaching at age forty-five. It is only too late if you never start! I feel timeless.

And happy. Last year, my first book, *Yoga Turns Back the Clock*, was published, and at the same time I got married to a wonderful and caring husband—a part-time cowboy with an East Texas ranch. Who could have imagined that a girl from South Africa would be living her dream in the American West! And now, with *Yoga Fights Flab*, my second book, I have achieved a level of success I could not have imaged just a decade ago.

But that success has less to do with any kind of monetary reward than it does with sharing the secrets of what I have learned with so many people. My program is not just for women, or just for men; it is not just for the thin, or the overweight; it is not just for the young, or the middle-aged. It is for everyone, no matter what your current level of fitness is. Yoga is, quite literally, something that can bring success to your life.

My heart was filled when I was able to write an acknowledgment in the book to my parents, knowing that they could finally relax and stop worrying about their little girl. I love you Mom and Dad Schneider.

Acknowledgments

You are what your deep, driving desire is.
As your desire is, so is your will.
As your will is, so is your deed.
As your deed is, so is your destiny.

         BRIDHADARANYAKA UPANISHAD

I feel honored to be able to thank so many people again, with this, my second book.

Jan Miller, my literary agent at Dupree Miller and Associates—you have the strength and power that anyone would admire. I owe you the deepest gratitude for your support and enthusiasm with this second project. Your sensitivity goes beyond the duties of an agent. I appreciate you so much!

Michael Broussard, my literary agent who creates with Jan at Dupree Miller—special friend first, agent second. You truly believe that what I do makes a difference, performing little miracles, always. You are supportive, generous with your time, and always willing to go that extra mile with me, with love from your "yoga goddess."

Kurt Twining, my beautiful, nurturing husband who walks the path of love with me—I know you are my number one fan, as I am yours. Your unconditional love and support in everything I do, no matter what turn it takes, helps me reach even higher!

My heartfelt thanks to my two beautiful daughters, Bodine Wolchuk and Kerry King, for your deep love and support, which are the basis for everything I do. Your total loyalty and immense enthusiasm magnify our deep love for one another.

Rockport Publishers and its associated company, Fair Winds Press—thank you for giving me the opportunity to write another book with you. I would like to express my love and gratitude to the following: Ken Fund, CEO; Holly Schmidt, Publisher; Amy DiGiovanni, North American Sales; Silke Braun, Art Director; Claire MacMaster, Design; Dalyn Miller, Marketing and Publicity Director; Donna Raskin, Acquisitions Editor; Brigid Carroll, Managing Editor; Rhiannon Soucy, Editorial Assistant; Janelle Randazza, Publicist; Jenny Beal, Photo Editor: for nurturing this book from conception to completion—you accomplish wonders. Silke, a special thanks to you for your professionalism and friendship. You are an absolute delight to work with.

Arnold Wayne Jones, friend, editor—Arn, your commitment to perfection, your infectious sense of humor, and your expertise were invaluable. Your professionalism and energy have brought this project to life. I am deeply grateful and honored to work with you.

World-class photographer Bobbi Bush and her assistant Tanya Fusco—I feel so fortunate to have you once again take all the beautiful photos for the book. You are such a pleasure to work with, it's not work—you make it easy and fun! Thank you for letting me be a part of your incredible work.

Deborah Coull and Lesley Griffin from Deborah Coull Salon and Aveda Concept and Sanctuary Salon—the second time working with you has been a true joy. Thank you for your creativeness in hair and makeup for the shoot. And thank you for the book signing at your store for *Yoga Turns Back the Clock*.

Thank you Anthony and Ellen Bolland for letting us set up a photo shoot every day at your beautiful property in Beverly Farms, Massachusetts, so we could get these wonderful photos for this book.

My mom and dad, Ann and Hyman Schneider—to you I owe the deepest gratitude. Your love is manifested in so many ways. Your sensitivity, love, and support throughout my life have opened the way for me and have kept it open against all odds. I thank you from the depths of my being. I have the most beautiful parents in the world. I love you both with all my heart.

Laura Diane Kurlansky, my sis, whom I lovingly call Lolly—miles have kept us away so many years, but you still are and always have been an inspiration to me. You have such strength—I thank you for your encouragement and love.

Mom and Dad, Vera and Lew Twining—Vera, you are the absolute living example of *Yoga Fights Flab*—I am so proud of you! You look absolutely wonderful and we have a testimonial in the book, too! Thank you! I am so fortunate to have you both in my life.

To Taylor, Cory, and Ryan Twining, thank you for your genuine caring, support, and encouragement—you are awesome.

A special thank you to world renowned Swami Isvarananda from the Sivananda Yoga School in Johannesburg, South Africa—your inspiration, guidance, and extended yoga knowledge challenged me to pursue my yoga practice to new heights.

To all my "yogis" and "yoginis" who come and spend such valuable time with me in class as we enjoy our sessions filled with passion and challenge together, and to all of you who are ready to fight the flab or get fit and stay fit—thank you for stepping onto this road where I have found the secret to living a healthy, strong, and vibrant life with many treasures and love.

About the Author

Glenda Twining is a yoga professional who lives and teaches in Dallas, Texas. She received her yoga certification from the Houston Institute under Lex Gillian, and extended yoga studies with Swami Yoga Sagar from the Bihar Yoga Bharati school and world-renowned Swami Isvarananda from the Sivananda Yoga school, both in Johannesburg, South Africa. She is a Physical Fitness Specialist and received such certification from the acclaimed Cooper Institute for Aerobics Research. She has studied extensively with teachers and gurus, both in the United States and abroad, and has helped orchestrate yoga retreats in the Yucatan.

The inspiration behind her teaching is to provide a balanced workout: A physiologically-based fitness regimen that promotes amazing weight loss results through increased cardiovascular, body strengthening, body sculpting and toning, flexibility, and increased emotional well-being. As this book demonstrates, she walks her talk.

Glenda's first book, *Yoga Turns Back the Clock*, was released in June 2003 to widespread acclaim as the first book of its kind to offer routines and information specifically tailored to exploring the anti-aging benefits of yoga. Glenda appears regularly in local media—newspapers, magazine articles, and on TV shows such as *Good Morning Texas*.

Glenda lives with her husband, Kurt. They divide their time between their Dallas home and an East Texas ranch.

A youthful woman of fifty-two, she credits her newfound youth, energy, and vigor—and her fit, lean, and muscular body—to her positive outlook and the yoga routines she practices daily, many of which are contained in this book.

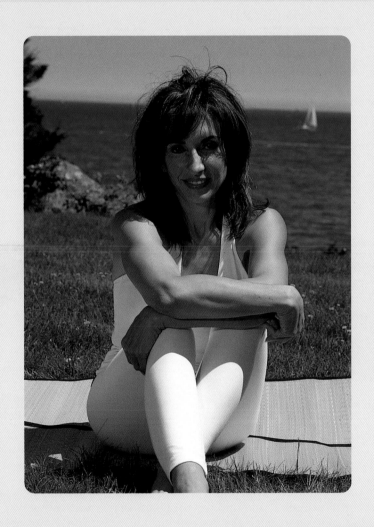

Also from Fair Winds Press

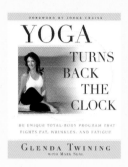

YOGA TURNS BACK THE CLOCK
By Glenda Twining
ISBN: 1-59233-006-1
$19.95 (£12.99)
Paperback; 192 pages
Available wherever books are sold

There Is a Magic Formula for Staying Young—Yoga!
You can be as toned, energized, and beautiful as you were in your twenties—or more so! Yoga practitioners have long known the secrets to looking and feeling young. Now you can harness the amazing power of this ancient art to rejuvenate every party of your body with the three energizing routines in this book.

Through simple step-by-step instructions and easy-to-follow full-color photos, Glenda Twining shows you the miracle of anti-aging yoga. She has helped hundreds of people turn back the clock with her unique program, and you can be next!

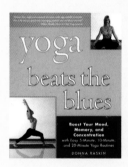

YOGA BEATS THE BLUES
By Donna Raskin
ISBN: 1-59233-022-3
$19.95 (£12.99)
Paperback; 176 pages
Available wherever books are sold

Feel Happier and More Relaxed in Minutes!
Yoga has been shown to reduce anxiety and improve symptoms of depression. In *Yoga Beats the Blues*, you'll learn simple yoga poses that clear the clutter in your mind and improve your outlook on life. These easy routines will help you feel better and release anxiety quickly. And, when practiced regularly, you can use these routines to keep depression and anxiety at bay forever.

With full-color photos and step-by-step instructions, Donna Raskin explains how to use yoga to improve your mood, relax, and find the happiness that resides within you. The routines are designed to take you through the day and include an early morning energizer, an afternoon mood pick-me-up, a relaxing evening routine, and numerous other poses and postures to encourage a calm and centered feeling.

You'll learn:
- Why yoga is a proven depression fighter and anxiety reliever
- What to do "on the spot" for a case of nerves or heartache
- How to calm yourself even if you're in a crowded room